Cut Short

I would like to dedicate this book to my rock and beautiful wife, Jose.

Cut Short

James Taylor

with

John Woodhouse

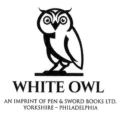

WHITE OWL

AN IMPRINT OF PEN & SWORD BOOKS LTD.
YORKSHIRE – PHILADELPHIA

First published in Great Britain in 2018 by
Pen & Sword White Owl
An imprint of Pen & Sword Books Ltd
Yorkshire - Philadelphia

Copyright © James Taylor, 2018

ISBN 9781526732378

The right of James Taylor to be identified as Author of this work
has been asserted by him in accordance with the Copyright,
Designs and Patents Act 1988.

A CIP catalogue record for this book is
available from the British Library.

Typeset in INDIA by Geniies IT & Services Private Limited

Printed and bound in the UK by TJ International

Pen & Sword Books Ltd incorporates the Imprints of Pen & Sword Books
Archaeology, Atlas, Aviation, Battleground, Discovery, Family History,
History, Maritime, Military, Naval, Politics, Railways, Select, Transport,
True Crime, Fiction, Frontline Books, Leo Cooper, Praetorian Press,
Seaforth Publishing, Wharncliffe and White Owl.

For a complete list of Pen & Sword titles please contact

PEN & SWORD BOOKS LIMITED
47 Church Street, Barnsley, South Yorkshire, S70 2AS, England
E-mail: enquiries@pen-and-sword.co.uk
Website: www.pen-and-sword.co.uk

or

PEN AND SWORD BOOKS
1950 Lawrence Rd, Havertown, PA 19083, USA
E-mail: us-pen-and-sword@casematepublishers.com
Website: www.penandswordbooks.com

Contents

Foreword

The decision to retire from professional sport is one of the toughest we face. It is a wonderful privilege to make a living from playing a game we love, but nevertheless, choosing the right time to quit is tricky. The danger is we leave it too long, desperately clinging to a lifestyle we do not want to let go, and become merely a shadow of the cricketer we once were. There is no right age to pack up. Graham Gooch, for example, scored twelve Test centuries and 4,500 runs after turning thirty-five, while I took the plunge into a new career aged thirty.

The point is that unless an injury comes along to spoil things, most of us can choose when to go and only very rarely is retirement from professional sport literally a choice between life and death. Yet that is the stark reality that confronted James Taylor in April 2016. He was twenty-six and, apparently, fit as a fiddle.

Geography demanded that I always took an interest in James's career. He was brought up in Burrough on the Hill on the Leicestershire border with Rutland, just a few miles from my home. I remember the excitement at Leicestershire County Cricket Club in 2008 when they secured his services, although inevitably his height (5' 6") prompted some discussion amongst the members. That Sachin Tendulkar at 5' 5" managed to score nearly 16,000 Test runs seemed to pass some by and besides, my experiences of bowling at short batsmen such as the West Indian left-hander Alvin Kallicharran (5' 4") inevitably ended unhappily: anything but intimidated by short-pitched fast bowling, they are ruthless cutters and pullers.

Those same members were left grumbling when, in 2012, James mirrored the hard-headed career move by Stuart Broad and transferred to Leicestershire's closest rivals, Nottinghamshire. In terms of ambition it was a no-brainer because Leicestershire had long vanished from the England selectors' radar and that is the fault of the system, not the players. Not only was James suggesting that he had an international future by scoring centuries for the England Lions, but he was also proving an effective leader. Indeed, before he was forced out of the game, I had seriously earmarked him as a prospective captain of England.

Ironically, I missed the first two days of James's Test debut against South Africa at Headingley because I was commentating on archery in the London Olympics. James showed great character in putting on 147 crucial first innings runs with Kevin Pietersen. The match was overshadowed by the revelation that Pietersen had sent messages about the captain, Andrew Strauss, to the South Africans, and had made disparaging comments about James's height. But James put all that to one side, earning respect as a man who clearly responds to a challenge.

As James departed with the squad for the 2015 World Cup in Australia, I bumped into a friend of Carol, his mother, in the local pub. A little fortified, I suspect, I suggested in no uncertain terms to her that at least one of the Taylors, who were unsure if he would be picked, should get themselves out to Melbourne to watch their son playing for England against Australia in the opening match of the tournament. The message was conveyed, and James's father Steve frantically booked last-minute tickets and arrived on the morning of the match.

I am so glad he was there, for this was an extraordinary spectacle. In the world's biggest cricket stadium, packed to the rafters with hostile Australian supporters, one of the world's smallest batsmen was bravely trying to avoid defeat to the old enemy. The cause was becoming increasingly hopeless, but James was playing a different game to the rest: my word, he batted well that evening. Chasing a massive 343 to win, England slumped to 92/6, but demonstrating his competitiveness, James hit 98 from 90 balls. No one else scored more than 37. A shambolic end resulted in the umpires incorrectly giving Jimmy Anderson run out and thereby denying James a certain century. I was commentating on the radio and was furious, but once again his character had caught the eye; and how proud his father must have felt.

In Cape Town the following year, Steve and Carol's timing was impeccable once again. This time they arrived in South Africa hours after James was out first ball in the New Year Test. This was a crucial series as James was given the chance to cement his place in the England Test team once more. Runs in Durban set him up, but just as crucial were some astonishing catches at short leg. Well, I say short leg. In fact, this was a careful placement of his own creation; deeper than usual to catch the ball from the full face of the bat. Typically, James had grasped the opportunity that fielding in the most unpopular position of all had presented and he set out to make himself the best in the business. He returned home firmly established as England's number five. Three months later, a potentially fatal heart condition forced him to retire.

The news shocked us all. I remember being so stunned that I could barely believe it. How, I wondered, would the fittest of young men who loved gym work, respond to being restricted to little more than pottering round the golf course?

Needless to say, James has confronted the situation head-on. We are thoroughly enjoying his company and his insight on the modern game on *Test Match Special*. I knew he would be good when, early on, he criticised a poor performance by his former Nottinghamshire teammates on air – never easily done. And I am assured that his golf has quickly become fiercely competitive. In fact, to borrow one of his words, he has become quite the badger.

Dealt a shattering blow, James Taylor's character is seeing him through. Frustratingly, after those memorable glimpses in Melbourne and South Africa, we will never know what might have been on the field, but he has already shown that there is no point dwelling on that. Instead, a talented, steely and engaging man is quickly showing us how much more he has to offer.

Jonathan Agnew MBE
Leicestershire
March 2018

Chapter 1

The End

By rights, I shouldn't be writing this book. I should have been found dead at the bottom of a flight of stairs. Or in the passenger seat of a car. Or on a cold wooden bench in a distant dressing room far from friends and family.

I might have died on my settee at home, or in front of a crowd of horrified onlookers in a hospital foyer. It sounds dramatic, but that's the black and white of it. People don't generally survive what I've come through. Eighty per cent of the time the condition that affects me is found in post-mortem. The first anyone knows a person has been suffering is when they're on the slab. Fair to say, my story could not have been written from the morgue.

If all had gone to plan, this book would have come after a long and illustrious international cricket career. It would have been peppered with tales of life in the England dressing room, of battles won and lost, of great opponents and even greater teammates. Maybe it would tell of a time I made an Ashes hundred, or saw England home to our first ever World Cup. For sure, if I was to have written an autobiography, I would never have expected an apparently innocuous early season game at Cambridge University to feature so highly. Certainly, in the big scheme of things, when my career was all wrapped up, as I'd imagined, in fifteen years time, I was never planning for this particular fixture to be anything other than a misty and distant memory. I had no idea that it would in fact be the one that would mark the end of my career and dictate my entire future life.

That journey down to Fenner's came after the longest time I'd ever had off in my whole career. While my Nottinghamshire teammates headed for preseason in the Caribbean, I stayed at home. Nothing against the Caribbean – normally I'd have lapped up the chance to escape the dreary last dregs of the English winter and feel the sun on my back in one of the most beautiful places on earth – but the truth was, I needed a break. Not a break because I was run down or injured or out of form. A break because I'd just had the most amazing non-stop winter with England, firstly in the United Arab Emirates to play Pakistan, and then South Africa, which had confirmed me as a regular in the England cricket team at Test as well as one day level. It was an ambition hard realised. A succession of ups and downs, pats on the back followed by kicks in the teeth. It was a path long and torturous, a route too often leading to dead ends of ill-informed opinion and, occasionally, prejudice against my size. Thankfully, I always had a never-ending drive and a close number of very special people to keep guiding the way, to take me over the next hurdle, and the next, and the next …

Nottinghamshire coach Mick Newell had allowed me to miss the preseason trip because he knew how hard I'd worked. Not only had I been away for months with England but I'd played much of the previous winter, firstly in Sri Lanka, and then a one day series down under followed by the World Cup in Australia and New Zealand, and then the full county season. Mick knew I needed a break and, let's face it, three weeks off wasn't much, especially if you were me – sitting still never came easy. Three weeks off for me wasn't like three weeks off for other people because I'd still be pushing myself relentlessly. In those three weeks, every single day I went to the gym. I did a lot of weights, which mentally and physically made me really strong. I had a mantra – 'Look good, feel good, play good' – and I loved smashing myself. I was compensating for a lack of height by getting myself as strong as I possibly could. When it came to making a statement of my ability on the pitch, I wanted max power.

At the same time, I had been feeling ill. I used to get colds a lot, probably because, without realising it, I was run down from training so hard and so much. I was on the edge of what my body could do all the time. Then I'd train through colds as well – the worst thing I could do – and that would tip me over into exhaustion. I was never good at giving myself proper down time even when I was supposedly having a rest.

Thankfully, I did do some chilling – I went two weeks without lifting a bat. Previously, if I hadn't picked a bat up for a week I might as well have been blindfolded when I eventually returned to the nets, but because now I knew my game so well I could pick it up and get straight back into it. And that's exactly what I did. I understood the areas I needed to concentrate on. I felt like I was getting my game down to a T.

When the 2016 season started, despite perhaps not resting quite as much as I might, I felt as physically and mentally strong as I'd ever been. It's not often as a professional sportsman you can say you have absolute clarity, but I had it then. After a run of five games in the England Test team I knew exactly what I needed to do to succeed in that form of cricket. Technically, I was in a great place, while in my head I was feeling liberated and light. Not only that, but to begin the summer, England were playing Sri Lanka at home. I knew I had an excellent chance of starting the series in the side and if ever there was a team to get runs against, it was Sri Lanka in England. They were a world-class side in their own backyard but outside of it they offered a real chance for England, and me, to start the summer in style.

Understandable, then, that I drove down to Cambridge the day before the game with not just hope, but expectation, in my heart. I slept well and next morning was up by 7.00 am doing yoga in bowler Harry Gurney's room. I wanted to give it a try as it's a good stretching exercise, as well as being brilliant for relaxation and loosening up – because I did so much gym I would get really stiff – so we set the iPad up and followed a simple routine.

Afterwards, I went down to eat. I always liked to have a good breakfast and this was no different – full English, with pain au chocolat, fruit and green tea, the only caffeine I ever had (I don't do normal tea or coffee), because I felt it was good for my metabolism.

By the time I'd eaten I felt fantastic. Here I was, a new season of excitement and opportunity ahead of me. All being well, this would be a chance to show what I was all about, a chance to confirm my place on the biggest stage of all, a chance to help win games for England. My time.

Cricket, though, as it's shown down the decades, doesn't like preordained plots and that day, after we won the toss and batted, I'd scored ten runs before I nicked off to second slip. I was disappointed because I wanted to spend some time at the crease. I felt so good. But the ball was swinging unbelievably and I got a nick on a wide half-volley. I was embarrassed, so frustrated – I couldn't believe I'd made the error. As I walked off I had no idea this would be my final innings. Caught Tom Colverd, bowled Connor Emerton. Between them they only ever played seven first class games of cricket.

Afterwards, I did some strength and conditioning work at the side of the pitch while watching Riki Wessels smash it to all parts. That was the way I was. If I wasn't batting, I'd be in the gym, or hitting balls. Just sitting was rarely on the agenda.

We were staying just outside Cambridge and that evening the team went for dinner at Yo! Sushi. I wasn't drinking, and so drove a few of the lads into town. It was just an average night, cricketers catching up and having a laugh, nothing to write home about, something that happens hundreds of times in a career.

After a decent night's sleep, next day was the same routine. Yoga with Harry, same breakfast, and then I drove myself to the ground. The England team had a sponsorship with Toyota and we all had Land Cruisers, one of the perks of being an international cricketer.

I arrived at Fenner's at 8.20 am and was in the nets for quarter to nine. I had a really good session with Nottinghamshire coach Peter Moores, apart from it being incredibly windy, to the extent that the nets, which were on wheels, were actually blown out of position. I helped the groundsman put them back into place before it started raining and I ran inside.

My immediate thought was, 'Thank God! It's raining! We're not going to have too much of a warm-up'. That's the mindset of a cricketer. They hate warming up. Sadly, it was only a shower and stopped after fifteen minutes, at which point we somewhat reluctantly ventured out. We went through our normal routine, playing volleyball football, where you use your feet to get the ball over the net instead of your hands, then it was standard mobility and agility routines, getting ourselves warm, before some light fielding practice – a few catches and throws.

I'd thrown five to ten balls when I started to feel a little bit anxious. My shoulder was sore – a hangover from the World Cup a year previously where it had been bothering me and causing me anxiety about throwing. Now I was anxious again. My chest started to feel tight. Out of nowhere, my heart was really thudding.

Everyone gets a little bit anxious – it's natural. But this was different. It felt beyond anxiety, like something had taken control of me and I couldn't do anything about it. I felt totally helpless. Anxiety usually subsides. This didn't. Right from the start it kept on going. It wasn't going to go away. I had ten seconds of feeling anxious. By fifteen I was turning to my teammate Brendan Taylor. 'My ticker's fucked,' I told him. 'My ticker's fucked.' Over and over again, I said it – 'My ticker's fucked. My ticker's fucked!'

My heart was now pounding like a drum – fast, loud, out of control. I felt breathless, panicky. My head was racing. 'Shit! What's happening to me?'

'Go and chill out, man,' Brendan advised. The warm-ups were coming to an end so I walked off to the changing rooms. My heart was now going what felt a million miles an hour. I could actually see my chest moving, my skin expanding and contracting, pulsing above my heart, fit to burst. It looked so unnatural. It made me feel sick to see it.

By the time I got into the changing rooms, I was really starting to sweat. It was a freezing cold April day but rivers were dripping from my face. I was so incredibly uncomfortable, like a stranger in my own skin. 'Fuck! Fuck!' again and again, was all I could think.

I lay down on the physio bed in the corridor – it's Cambridge, the facilities aren't the greatest. I was still sweating like anything. By now, whatever was happening to me had been going on for two minutes and I was really struggling to breathe. I was gasping for air, sucking it in. I was feeling so, so sick. I slumped off the physio bed, made it into the toilet and stuck my head in the pan, desperately trying to vomit. Nothing would come. Nottinghamshire physio Jon Alty dragged me out of there. It hadn't been flushed and was no place for anyone to be putting their face. He got me back on the physio bed. I was trying to tell him about my heart but I could barely breathe. Every intake of air was a massive effort. I was gulping it in. I thought I was going to die.

I just wanted it to stop. I was so cold, really cold, but sweating at the same time. My heart was still banging at what to me felt like a million miles an hour. I wanted to pass out. I was willing myself to pass out. That would be a way of escaping it. I was thinking, 'What will it feel like to pass out?' I'd never done it before. I wanted now to be the moment I found out, but that particular relief never came.

Alty fetched me a drink but I was shaking so much that I couldn't hold it and dropped it on the floor.

At this stage the lads were going out to field. They saw me but thought nothing of it. They just thought I was feeling a bit offside. They also might have thought I was trying to get out of fielding. Sounds harsh, but if I'd seen someone else in my position, a bit of me would have thought exactly the same. A lot of people don't like fielding, let alone in early April against a university side in the cold.

At the same time, in the sporting world, showing any sign of weakness is not the done thing. I probably held back from saying what I was really feeling, and that may have influenced how everyone in that dressing room perceived what was happening. Hindsight is a wonderful thing, but at that point I had no reason to think I was in the grip of something truly horrific. In my head, this was something temporary that I just needed to grit my teeth and get through. I guess I felt a little self-conscious about pressing the panic button too publicly. I was at the start of experiencing an earthquake but was probably trying to give the impression it was a tremor.

Even so, I couldn't help the odd moment of panic. 'I can't breathe! I can't breathe!' I spluttered at one point.

Riki Wessels popped up. 'Don't worry, Phys,' he told Alty. 'I've seen this in a film. You just stab a pen in his throat to create another air hole.'

It was a bit of black humour – except a bit closer to the knuckle than Riki might have thought. At that point I really did think I was on the way out. A biro through the neck wasn't out of the question where I was sitting.

Eventually, the players left and Alty gave me a sugary drink because he thought I might be suffering a shock reaction to low blood sugar levels. He was asking what I had for breakfast. He wanted to give me oxygen but even in the state I was in I was aware that the corridor was a bit public. My body was in breakdown but my head was still working really well and I was conscious that I didn't want anyone to see me like this.

I went next door into the cold dark changing rooms and as I lay down on the hard wooden slats of the benches, propped against the wall, Alty gave me oxygen. While I lay there, he spoke on the phone to an England doctor. I was really battling now. My head was telling me again and again I was in a serious situation. My heart felt like it was running away with itself but more than that it was irregular and out of rhythm. That was the key for me. That was what frightened me. It was so irregular, so fast, and so incredibly uncomfortable. Physically seeing your shirt moving is scary. As a kid growing up you think your heart is in the left-middle of your chest and that if you could see it beat that would be where it would show. And yet here I was, and now it was beating out the side of my body. Before, no matter how hard I pushed myself, I'd never felt my heart hit the wall. I'd feel it beating, of course, just like anyone would. Now it felt like someone was physically punching me from the inside, their fist visible in my chest.

Subconsciously, I was thinking the oxygen was going to help, same with the sugary drinks. The placebo effect, I think they call it. Whatever, I was feeling a fraction better. And at that point, that was a major leap forward for me.

Alty was describing the symptoms to the ECB doctor, and the feedback he was getting from the symptoms I was describing and the demeanour I was giving out was that it could be a viral illness and that I should be monitored. It was a strange situation. The truth is that at times I genuinely thought I was going to die, and my heart was smashing through my chest, but I'm obviously no medical expert and I was happy to go along with the idea of a virus – all I wanted was this whole horrible situation to go away.

I was on the oxygen for twenty to thirty minutes but didn't move from the bench for almost an hour. Alty checked my pulse by hand and also put a pulse oximeter on the end of my finger to check my vital signs. My pulse reading was up from normal but not off the scale. But to me this wasn't a bit of kit equipped to deal with whatever else was happening in my body. I kept looking at this little plastic machine. I kept saying it felt a lot worse than this little bit of information it was chucking out. 'Fuck what it says,' I said, 'feel my heart!'

Ross Herridge, our strength and conditioning coach, came and did just that. This stupid little machine was still saying the situation wasn't as bad as I was feeling. So there we were, all under the assumption it was probably a virus. I had no reason to suppose anything different. I was a young man at the peak, or so I thought, of physical fitness. I had no reason to kick up a fuss, and I didn't.

The idea was that I should stay at the game and see how I went in the next few hours. In the meantime, an appointment was made for me to see the Nottinghamshire team doctor back in Nottingham. It wouldn't be anytime soon. He was working in Leicester and would have to finish his daily rounds before he travelled to Nottingham to see me. I wouldn't be seeing him before 6.00 pm.

Then, as the coaches went out to assess various matters happening in the game, I was left on my own. Just me, an empty dressing room, and my hideous discomfort. All the time, I couldn't believe how uncomfortable I felt. I must have tried ten different places in the changing room to lie down, or sit, or prop myself up. I lay on benches. I lay in the showers. I lay on the floor. But this was Fenner's, not Lord's. Relief was thin on the ground. The floor was concrete, cold, even more so since I'd been sweating so much that my clothes were wet. The benches were wooden slats. I was using people's clothes, pads, anything to lie on, to give myself at least a slight degree of comfort. It was like when you have a really bad hangover, or feel unendingly nauseous, that sheer level of discomfort. Generally, in those situations you end up in the foetal position, but whatever position I tried nothing changed. To be comfortable I needed to take off my skin.

Just before twelve, I rang my girlfriend (now wife) Jose. It was the Easter holidays and, a teacher, she'd driven to Shropshire from our home in Nottingham to see her family. I needed to speak to somebody, and there was never anyone better than Jose. She has always reassured me in times of need and always will.

'There's nothing wrong,' I told her. 'There's nothing to worry about.' If ever there's a way to alert someone that something serious is going on, that's it. Straight away she knew. Before I'd even explained she could tell from my voice. I was fainter than usual, still struggling to breathe.

'It's my heart,' I told her. 'It's racing, going up and down. It's going mad.'

Jose knows me better than I do. To say we're close doesn't come near. She knows me inside out. She was trying her best to find out exactly what was happening. I was doing my best to talk, but at the same time I was so uncomfortable. I needed to get off the phone. I needed to be quiet. I didn't have it in me to speak anymore. I didn't have it in me to do anything other than try to deal with what was happening to me. I was conscious as well of not wanting to worry her. Maybe the less I said the better.

'I've got to go,' I said, and put the phone down.

Eventually, I made my way upstairs to the viewing area in the bar. I was still incredibly uncomfortable but thought it might divert me a little from how I was feeling. I was sipping at drinks and also tried to eat a banana but couldn't manage it as I felt so sick.

I then tried to have a walk outside with Alty to watch a little bit of the game from closer quarters. I was incredibly cold, even when I put a hoodie on, and yet was sweating like anything. I was feeling just awful. I could speak and hold a conversation, anything to take my mind off how awful I felt, but I could never escape the pitiless grip of whatever was happening inside me.

There was clearly no way I was going to play and it was thought best if I headed home in the lunch interval. I obviously wasn't fit to drive and there was nobody who could take me back to Nottingham apart from the overseas player, Aussie bowler Jackson Bird. Jackson wasn't playing, but that didn't mean we could set off back straight away. It was deemed he had to have a practice bowl in the middle, and lunch was the only time the pitch would be free. It's hard to overstate how desperate I was to get out of there and get home, just lie on my settee, clamber into bed, just find a little bit of comfort, and now here I was, having to wait even longer for the overseas player to have a bowl. I had no other choice but to go along with it – I had no one else to take me home.

As Jackson went out, the other guys came back in. There might usually have been a bit of piss-taking but they could see I wasn't winging it. Instead it was just typical blokes.

'Are you all right, mate?"

'Yeah, just feeling a bit rough.'

Again, I was just palming them off, trying to disguise how bad my heart was. I didn't want them to know what I really felt like inside. It's professional sport – the changing room isn't a place where you show weakness. I even sat upstairs in the dining area with them for a bit and then went back downstairs to try to get comfortable again.

Eventually, Jackson finished his session and we walked to his BMW. I'm usually pretty precious about my belongings but that day I couldn't have cared less. I left my bags unpacked in the changing room and abandoned my car. The only thing I took was my phone. All I could think was, 'I've got to get out of here'.

I didn't know Jackson at all. We had literally met that day. It was a two-hour drive to Nottingham and as I slumped against the window in the passenger seat, I apologised for being antisocial. I was in no fit state to hold a conversation. I turned my head and rested on the seatbelt and tried to get as comfortable as I could. Rest wasn't easy. There was no respite in my heart. It was still pounding away. But it was just as much the irregularity as the pounding. It was the most awful feeling. Like a wrecking ball smashing against a wall. Except that wrecking ball was my heart and that wall was me.

The movement of the car allowed me brief escape from the torture as it induced a short fifteen-minute sleep. About twenty-five minutes out from Nottingham, however, I woke up with a start.

'Shit. I've got no house keys.'

In my desperation to get out of there, I'd left them at Cambridge. It was just something else to add to an already dreadful mix. I tried to contact my neighbour because she had a spare set, but with no joy. I then rang my mum, who only lived half an hour away. Up until then, I hadn't bothered to tell my parents something was wrong.

'Mum, I'm really ill,' I told her. 'I've had to come back from Cambridge. I haven't got my keys. Can you bring me your spare set?"

Mum wasn't hugely surprised to hear of my predicament. She'd always followed my career closely and noticed online straight away that I hadn't started the game that morning. Also, Jose had rung her and told her something was amiss. I wasn't in the mood to chat and so just told her I'd meet her at Trent Bridge.

'Please,' I told her, 'be as quick as you can.'

Jackson dropped me outside the ground and I clambered out of his car. I was in a hell of a state, but also I'm a bloke so I was trying not to give too much away. I didn't want anyone to see me in such a mess. 'I've got to man up here,' I chided myself. I was quite literally dying inside – but I couldn't possibly let anyone see that.

It was a Wednesday in early April. There was nothing going on at Trent Bridge. The only people there were the office ladies, and, lovely as they were, I didn't really feel like going to say hello to them. 'Hi! I'm dying! How's things with you?'

I just needed to get inside the pavilion and get my head down again. I curled up at the bottom of the stairs to the lunch room. As I lay there, I must have made for a piteous sight. Just a few weeks earlier I'd been scoring runs and taking miracle catches for England in South Africa. Now I was a hunched, grey, hollow figure on the verge of death.

Fifteen minutes I lay there, and it's hard not to think that my mum could well have found me dead. The newspaper headlines would have reflected something far different from the 'plucky retirement' narrative they would soon be declaring in the sports pages.

My mum had never negotiated the corridors of the pavilion but somehow found me in a ball at the foot of those stairs. She was shocked to see how ill I was and, like any mum, her first instinct was to look after me. She took me home, just half a mile up the road, and I staggered through the door before lying down on the settee on my left side. It was a big soft comfy sofa, and yet that whole settee was vibrating, with my every heartbeat going deep into the furnishings. The sound was horrendous, to the point that I couldn't stand it anymore and turned on to my right side.

Mum wanted to take me to hospital but because of what I'd been told at Cambridge, and believed myself, that it was just a virus, my mindset was still that I just needed to battle through. 'Give it a day and I'll be OK,' I was telling myself. 'I can't feel like this tomorrow.' My mum put blankets on me because I was still really cold. All the time she was wanting to take me to hospital, but again and again I was saying no.

After hearing me on the phone and speaking to my mum, Jose had made the decision to come home straight away. My mum met her at the door and the first thing she said to her was, 'Go in and feel his heart.' I got up off the sofa and Jose came towards me. When she put her hand on my heart I could see how shocked she was. There was almost a physical recoil. She wanted to take me to hospital straight away, but I refused, so dominant was talk of a virus in my head. In any case, I was meant to be seeing the doctor at 6.00 pm and by now it was four in the afternoon. It didn't seem that long to wait.

I could hear Jose and my mum having a discussion in the kitchen about calling an ambulance. By now I'd been on the sofa about half an hour. As I was trying, and failing, to get comfortable, I was feeling progressively worse, like I was going to be sick. I was also getting pains in my left shoulder and down my left arm. I was thinking, 'This is strange – I haven't been to the gym. I haven't done a proper session for two days. Why am I so achy in my shoulder?' Looking back, it's obvious – most people know if you get a pain in your shoulder it's the sign of a heart attack. Not me, though. Not at that moment. My remedy was to try to give myself a bit of a massage. It didn't last long, my body was collapsing inside. I knew I had to go and be sick.

I made it to the bottom of the stairs but didn't have the energy to walk up. Instead I shuffled up on my hands and knees. At the top of the landing was the toilet. I crawled in and was sick repeatedly, five times. I shouldn't have been alive at that stage. With my body concentrating all it had on my vital organs, my stomach was already giving up. I felt so terrible – pain, nausea, my heart smashing out of my chest – that going back downstairs wasn't an option. Across the landing was my bed. It had to be the warmest and most comfortable place to be. I crawled in and pulled the duvet over me. It wasn't the relief I was hoping for. My heart was still pounding, flying, hammering in my chest. My shoulder was still really sore.

As my body directed my blood to the real areas of emergency, my hands and feet were freezing. My mum was making a hot water bottle downstairs while Jose came up to me. She rang the doctor from by my bed. He was still on his rounds in Leicester. There was no way he was going to make it for 6.00 pm. Jose described my symptoms – the sickness, the fast and irregular heartbeat, the pains in the shoulder. He didn't hesitate. 'Take him straight to hospital. Don't wait for an ambulance. Just go.'

By this time, Dad had rung. An ex-jockey, he's now a race starter and that day he happened to be working at Nottingham racecourse. As soon as he heard what was happening, he knew straight away what needed to happen – 'Get him straight to hospital!'

I hauled myself out of bed, down the stairs and into the back of mum's car with Jose. Whenever mum's driving, Jose and I always jump in the back, and this, although in slightly different circumstances, was no different. Jose had grabbed loads and loads of coats off the pegs as well as a blanket, and somewhere underneath them all was me. The Queen's Medical Centre was only ten minutes away in the car but mum didn't know the way. I wouldn't have known either had I not had to run a plumber there a few weeks earlier after he'd sliced his thumb open on a ceramic tile while working on our shower.

Mum dropped us outside A&E and Jose and I walked up to reception.

'I think we're going to have blag this a bit so they know I'm poorly,' I told her. 'I need to see someone. I don't want to be sat around for two hours.'

When we're together, Jose does all the talking and this was exactly the same. She was speaking to the receptionist, explaining what was going on. I knew I was going to be sick again. Luckily there was a toilet straight behind me. I staggered in, threw up, came back out, went to reception, and then dived straight back into the loo to be sick again. I was sick repeatedly until nothing more could come. It's odd, but while I felt like I was dying physically, I still had some mental awareness about me. I was conscious of being an England cricketer; this was a busy hospital and some people might know who I was. There was a bit of me that didn't want people to see me being sick, to see me in such a bad condition. I was trying my best to look normal. I expect I looked far from it.

As I came out of the toilet the second time, a doctor walked past and saw me. By this time I was grey. All the blood had drained from my face. It was clear something was seriously wrong. She immediately took me and

Jose into a little assessment room nearby. Our anxiety was bursting from every vein. 'Calm down, calm down,' she said. 'I'll just do an ECG.' She lifted my top, put the pads and wires on my chest and took a look at the screen. I didn't see her face but I knew something fairly remarkable was happening. More doctors were called and when they saw the results, that was it – they took me straight through to where the real action happens, a more serious setup, a big cubicle – resus. There were wires, machines, everywhere.

They sat me up at a 45 degree angle on a hospital trolley and immediately hooked me up to a heart monitor. The sound it made was like nothing you'll ever hear. A cavalcade of beeps, fast – faster than fast – ricocheting around the room. It was the sound of my heart. Loud. Everybody could hear it. It was charging, careering, thundering. A runaway train trapped within my ribs. The machine said it was pounding away at 265 beats a minute.

The doctors looked at one another. Strangely, it's the little things you notice at a time like that, and the expression on their faces – shock, disbelief – is something I won't forget in a hurry. More and more medics were flooding in. They closed the curtains, and took my top off, inserting a cannula, taking blood and hooking me up to a drip. There were people coming in and out all the time. It was so busy.

Physically I was gone, but mentally I was still switched on. Even as things were kicking off in the hospital room when they were trying to save me, I could still think on my feet.

'He's slurring his words,' stated a nurse.

'I'm always like this,' I replied. 'You want to hear me on a bad day.'

On the other hand, I was clearly befuddled – it was the first time I can remember where I took off my top without thinking about my six-pack.

The blood results came back at record speed. When the heart is under stress it releases an enzyme called troponin. Under no stress, the amount of troponin in the blood would be zero. My level was 42,000. It was extraordinary. Unsurprisingly, at that point they concluded I'd had a severe heart attack, because the stress my heart was under was just phenomenal.

First priority was to get my heart out of its abnormal rhythm. 'There are two options,' they told me. 'We pump you full of drugs and hopefully that works, and if it doesn't, we put you to sleep and shock you out of it.'

I didn't like the sound of the second one. I was adamant the drugs were going to work. There was no way I was going to be shocked. I couldn't bear the thought of those big metal pads being placed against me, sending up to a thousand volts coursing through my body.

Me being me, I was thinking positive. 'Well, if the drugs work,' I told Jose, 'there'll be no need for them to shock me. They'll work; it'll be fine.'

And yet after the drugs were administered, nothing happened. Minutes ticked by. All we could do was wait. Panic rapidly rising. All the time that awful sound of the machine in the corner racing. It appeared my positivity had been misplaced.

Jose was urging me to have the shock instead. 'You'll feel so much better afterwards,' she reassured me. 'Just do it. You're going to feel amazing. You'll go right back to normal. It's just a tiny thing and then you'll feel better.'

But I was so scared. The only time I'd seen a defibrillator used was on TV programmes where they were a last resort, something to bring people back from the dead. I used to watch *Casualty* a lot when I was younger, and when things went wrong, out came the pads. In the end, they called the anaesthetist through to put me to sleep. It seemed my worst nightmare was coming true. And then, a matter of seconds before the anaesthetist arrived in the room, there was a massive change. Like a lift down a shaft, my heart rate plunged. In a matter of seconds it went from 265 to 60. The machine in the corner was making a different noise – a steady 'beep, beep, beep', where before it had been manic. It was the best noise I'd ever heard. One of the best feelings I've ever had. I'll never forget it. It sounds daft but it really felt like we were celebrating. Jose and I had been holding hands the whole time and now it felt like we'd crossed the winning line together. Whatever it was, we'd beaten it.

And then I was sick everywhere.

My heart might have been back to 'normal' but the rest of my body was completely screwed. It had put everything into saving my heart. That meant other areas had suffered. I was a matter of seconds from my kidneys failing and my entire digestive system had pretty much stopped. But I was feeling better. Rough, obviously, but not nearly as uncomfortable as I had been. All I'd wanted for the last seven hours was for the horribleness, the hideous agony and overwhelming anxiety of my heart beating its violent rhythm, the feeling that I was being overtaken by something, potentially deathly, out of my control, to stop. And now it had.

At that point my dad arrived. He didn't say anything – even now, we've never really spoken about it – but to see me in that situation, surrounded by medical equipment, dozens of staff, the noise, the bustle, must have been a shock.

Medical personnel seemed to be swarming in from all sides to make further investigations. One of them asked, 'How did you get here?'

'We just drove in.'

'No, how did you get into this room?'

'We just walked in.'

'No, you don't understand. How did you get in here, into A&E, where we are now?'

Jose said again: 'We walked in.'

'You walked in here?' I don't think she thought we were thinking straight. 'That's impossible. You couldn't have. Not like this.'

An Asian doctor who liked his cricket spoke up. 'I know who he is,' he declared. 'I saw him. He just walked in here. He came straight in.'

One of the doctors stood there open-mouthed. 'It's remarkable.'

They asked how long I had been suffering. 'It started about half past ten this morning.'

'What?' It was utter astonishment. 'What you've been through is the equivalent of running six marathons.'

My sheer fitness had saved me. Anyone else wouldn't have had a chance. It was now five o'clock. I'd been like this for six and a half hours. Most people who go through what I'd gone through are passed out after ten minutes.

A doctor tried to explain: 'We think you've had a little event.'

I didn't know what he meant. I wished he'd just said 'heart attack', because that was what I thought he was alluding to.

'An event?' I was confused. 'What do you mean?'

'Well,' he continued, 'you know Fabrice Muamba?'

I knew Fabrice Muamba. He was the former Bolton Wanderers midfielder who 'died' on the pitch during a game against Tottenham Hotspur at White Hart Lane. His heart stopped for seventy-two minutes. By rights there was no way he should have been alive. He was, quite literally, the man who came back from the dead.

Inside I sunk. 'Oh God.' But at the same time I was thinking, 'Well, I'm here. I'm still standing. Yes, I've had an "event", but I haven't "died" like he did. Yes, what's happened is terrible, but my heart hasn't stopped. I've managed OK – I've made it through.'

In fact, at that point, I was getting ready to go home. That was it, as far as I was concerned. All over. Done. But when everything had calmed down a little, the doctors told me I would need to stay in. 'Really? Stay in hospital overnight? Come on!'

It sounds ridiculous, I know, but my only thought was I needed to be ready in three weeks' time for the home series with Sri Lanka. That was what I was saying to the doctors. So when they were telling me I needed to stay for a night, or two, or three, I was saying, 'No, no – I've got to get out of here. I need to be ready for then.'

I kept asking them over and over if I really had to stay in hospital. It was all that was in my head. And remember, this is at a time when I could well have been dead. But that's where I was with it. That's how little idea I had of just how serious the whole thing was. To my mind, I'd had a problem, they'd sorted it out, and now it was time to go home and carry on with my life. I'd quite happily have disappeared there and then, but they were insistent. They told me they were going to transfer me over to the City Hospital, which has a specialist cardiac unit.

And that's what they did. Before I knew it, they'd strapped me in an ambulance, lights flashing, sirens on. This time, we couldn't travel in the back together – Jose was in the front. On arrival, I was whizzed inside and straight into a medical room. There were literally fifteen doctors and ambulance staff in there. They all seemed to think I'd had a heart attack and were telling me what they needed to do to see what was going on. Echocardiogram, angiogram – they were just words at the time, but we know what they are now. There was even talk of me needing surgery that night, but thankfully some more test results came through. An emergency operation wasn't necessary.

When the cardiologist came in, a trainee doctor who'd travelled with us from the first hospital had to report to him. 'We think he's had a heart attack,' he said. 'He needs an angiogram.'

The consultant took one look at him. 'He's had a heart rate of 265 for six hours, there's no way he had a heart attack.' My heart simply couldn't have sustained it. This was something completely different. 'He doesn't need an angiogram.'

My body was in a state, but again, my head was so good that I was conscious of feeling sorry for the doctor. He was a trainee. Originally, I'd thought, 'Do not let that person look after me if he's not trained.' And then I felt really bad because he was such a lovely guy. He knew I played cricket for England and by the time we got to the second hospital he'd been with us practically from the start. In mine and Jose's eyes, he'd saved my life.

Of course, just because I didn't need an angiogram didn't mean they wouldn't need to do other investigations. For now, though, they took me to my own room upstairs. It was 7.00 pm. The last nine hours had been a blur. A day that should have been so anonymous had turned out, for all the wrong reasons, to be one I would never, could never, forget. It had begun twelve hours previously with me doing yoga in Harry Gurney's room. Ironically, yoga, of course, is meant to chill you out. And yet, no sooner had I started doing it than this had happened! Ban all yoga!

Mum and Dad stayed with me for a while but eventually they headed off. It had been a hell of a day for me, but for them as well. A day that had started like any other had ended up with them facing their son nearly dying. I've no idea what that must feel like for a parent and I hope I never have to find out.

In the room, there was this lovely nurse, so welcoming. 'Can I get you any food?' she asked.

I'd eaten nothing all day and didn't really want anything – it felt like I'd been sick a million times. All I could think of was my go-to as a kid, and even now when I can't be bothered cooking.

'I don't suppose you've got any tomato soup?'

She went off to have a look. 'Would Heinz be OK?'

'Oh my God! Brilliant!' At last things were looking up.

Jose didn't want to leave me – actually, it was more than that; wild horses wouldn't have dragged her away from my bedside, but the first night she was worried she wouldn't be able to remain outside visiting hours.

'Can I stay?' she asked the nurse, firmly expecting the answer to be 'no'. 'Just this one night, please?'

'Yes, of course you can stay,' said the nurse. It wasn't exactly luxury on offer – just the cold hard floor of my room. All she had was a pillow and a blanket. But she would be there next to me, and that's all that mattered to both of us. It was an early sign of the absolute strength and devotion she would reveal in the days, weeks, months and years to come.

Emotionally, I'd kept everything in check for the whole day. As I lay down to sleep, though, it all became too much for me. The day, my heart, the future – there were so many unanswered questions, so much to deal with. It was the first time I'd ever felt real fear. Raw unbridled fear. Jose lay next to me and I held her close.

'This isn't good,' I whispered. 'When are we going to get out of here?'

She no more had the answer than I did. Her life had been tipped upside down, shaken around, and she'd come hurtling into this strange new world just the same as me.

'We've still got me and you,' she hugged me, 'and that's all that matters.' She said it again and again. 'Nobody has what we have.'

I lay there still in the same Nottinghamshire emblazoned training kit I'd been wearing when I'd first felt my heart go haywire. At that point it never occurred to me that I might never wear it, or the three lions of England, again.

Looking further down the bed, I noticed I even had the same socks on from the start of the day. Two left socks – a bad luck sign if ever there was one.

I'll never do that again.

Chapter 2

The Start

My parents always say I never watched TV. It's one of the reasons I didn't have any sporting heroes growing up. I was always too busy doing something. Generally, that meant being outside. And generally, that meant some kind of sport-related activity.

We were lucky to have a couple of fields at the back of the house I could mess about in, or I'd mark out football pitches in the garden. I was pretty creative. I put together some home-made rugby posts so I could learn to kick, and I was always playing tennis against a wall, hitting golf balls, or trying to find the middle of the basketball net. Wherever I went I'd take a tennis ball with me, always throwing it against a wall, practising my catching. That natural hand-eye co-ordination that would serve me so well came from that constant playing, throwing, hitting and catching. Over time I then added ability, agility, speed and awareness. I would find ways of achieving what I wanted, be it scoring a goal from a ridiculous angle or snaffling a lightning-quick rebound off a wall down low. I always found a way to get something done. I could adapt, find a way forward, and without realising it I was giving myself skills that would put me way ahead of most other kids my age. Maths, I was never that good at, but give me an angle on a sports pitch and I'd be all over it. Strip most sports back and you have to know angles down to a T. That's sporting knowledge, not academic.

Home was Burrough on the Hill, in the part of Leicestershire that forms a patchwork of green fields and muddy lanes peppered with pretty and very typically English villages. It sounds idyllic, and it was. But there weren't a great deal of other kids to do much with. Instead I spent a lot of time by myself. I have a sister, Sarah, but she's two years older than me and all we did as kids was fight. We couldn't play tennis together because we'd whack each other instead of the ball. If we were around the stables, we'd even use horse whips! Horses were a big part of Taylor life. I got on a horse as soon as I could walk – before I had hair even – and there's a fading family photo of me, aged just two, stood up on the back of a pony. It was inevitable. My dad was a jockey, whilst my sister rode for Great Britain Juniors and my mum was also no slouch in the saddle, winning a few point-to-point races.

Sport, then, was massive for me from infancy. It was what I knew, what I loved, but my parents wanted me to have an education as well. They thought they could combine the two, and add a bit of discipline into the mix, by sending me to boarding school at Maidwell Hall, 30 miles away in Northamptonshire. In fact, it was because of discipline that they sent me a term early before the summer break. They reckoned I'd been a bit naughty at my old school, Brooke Priory, in Oakham, where Stuart Broad's mum was a teacher, and possibly they were right. I'd soon realised I could get sent out of lessons for talking too much or messing about. I didn't see that punishment as much of a deterrent. From where I was sitting, bored to tears in the classroom, the corridor was a much better option. Maidwell, though, was different. If I misbehaved there, they'd say, 'Right, no sport.' I didn't like that at all.

As an 8-year-old, I was homesick at first. I used to have really bad nightmares, waking up not knowing where I was, and the son of a family friend in the top year would look after me. I began sleepwalking as well. Once, back at home, when my parents had gone out, I sleepwalked down the stairs, past the babysitter, out the front door, along the drive, and down the road. I was screaming for my mum. I ended up knocking on a neighbour's door, and that's when I woke up. They took me back home. Imagine the babysitter's face!

There is always an assumption that it's somehow odd for children to go to boarding school as young as eight. But, while I had that bout of homesickness early on, I never thought there was anything unusual or unlikeable about it. My mum had gone to boarding school so there was a tradition of it in the family, and it was what I had always expected to do. As well as that, my parents would often be there watching me play one sport or another, so there wasn't as big a separation as some might think.

Boarding school also helped me to discover the real me. It toughened me up massively, instilled an independent spirit, and made me mentally strong. That's why, when I got older, I never minded touring, because I was so used to being away from home. It also taught me the mechanics of being around the same group of people day in, day out. I was sleeping in a room with eight other lads, and, at a very young age, you have to work that out and find the best way forward. It's a complex mixture of getting on with people and fending for yourself. Boarding school is a tough atmosphere if you're not enjoying it. But soon enough, I did enjoy it, and a lot of that was because I'd worked out the pattern of cogs – social, sporting and otherwise – that made it work.

Once I'd settled in, I loved school. Maidwell Hall was made for sport. It had massive grounds and was very much based on an outdoor lifestyle. I got to play sport every day with my mates – it doesn't get much better than that – and I began to see it as home. Rugby and football were the big ones for me. As well as playing both at Maidwell, I played rugby for nearby Oakham and football at Melton Mowbray. I lived for scoring tries at rugby and goals at football. It was all I cared about.

Cricket entered the equation when we went on holiday. My mum's aunt had a lovely house at Sandilands, near Skegness, and for three weeks every summer we'd pack up a horse trailer and two cars and head off. The house had a big garden, and that was without the massive expanse of beach nearby – perfect for cricket. It was a sport that was rapidly seeping into my life. At Maidwell, there was a proper cricket structure, with the school playing other teams. Every Wednesday and Saturday, we had a match and in between we'd train. My entire life revolved around sport. A family friend asked me what I played in the summer – 'cricket' – what I played in the winter – 'football' – and which was my favourite – 'rugby'.

It was at Maidwell that I met Steve Schofield, the cricket coach who would have such a huge influence on me and my career. Not that it started off particularly well. Our first encounter was in the indoor school during a game of Kwik cricket. Players were meant to rotate round the field but I wouldn't move. Steve wasn't impressed. 'What's your name, young man?'

'James Taylor.' He wasn't going to forget it.

Steve will openly admit that at first he found me irritating. I'd taken my habit of carrying a ball around with me, bouncing it off the walls, to Maidwell. Except now I didn't have just one, I had several. Steve would confiscate one, but I had a pocketful, and two minutes later I'd be doing it again.

I was a very busy child and would get bored easily. I had to be doing something. If someone was playing football, I'd walk into the game and join in. But even at that age I needed something to aim at – still do now. If I went in goal at football in the gym at lunchtime, I wouldn't pass to my mates – I'd roll it out, run the length of the pitch, and try to score. It was the same with rugby. I wouldn't pass; I'd try to score the tries myself. I was very competitive. I just wanted to win.

Cricket, though, was different – because Steve made it different. 'If you're going to do this,' he told me, 'you've got to do it my way.' I still loved other sports but cricket became much more defined. At that point, if my parents had thought I was destined for a sporting career, then they'd have been thinking rugby or football, but Steve said to my dad straight away, 'Don't discount cricket.' He developed me for the long term. 'Keep the game simple,' was his mantra. 'Get your base right and everything else follows.' My head was still, my base was still, and I had quick hands and feet. The building blocks of success were all there.

The whole way through my sporting life I've always had mentors, and Steve was the first. He had great cricket connections, working in youth development with Leicestershire County Cricket Club, and could see the promise in me from an early age. At just nine, for instance, he got me in at Loughborough Town CC. 'He'll play for England,' he told the coach. They could see my potential too.

Straight away I was playing with lads aged fifteen. Aged twelve, I played for the men's team. That's where it started – the love of going in, building an innings, and scoring big runs. That experience would have a long-lasting effect. As I moved onwards and upwards, I was never fazed by being in teams with older lads. In fact, if anything, it felt like I got on with them better than with lads of my own age.

Also, while I was a 'posh boarding school boy', at Loughborough Town maybe two out of twenty lads went somewhere similar. The rest were from all sorts of different backgrounds and I loved being among a mix of people rather than staying in one particular group. A lot of kids from my background get stuck with turning their noses up at other people, but I was lucky enough to avoid that fate, and so much of that came from playing sport with a wide range of characters. I can't overestimate how important that was. Building relationships and learning to fit in and adapt is a skill that everybody needs, both in cricket and in life. From a very early age I was used to playing for new teams, playing with different age groups. I had nothing to fear from changing environments. I embraced change rather than shunned it.

That confidence came from Steve driving me forty-five minutes every Saturday to Loughborough. If he didn't take me, his wife Nikki would. They'd taken a shine to me early on – fortunately the cheekiness and boundless energy was as endearing as it was irritating – and they went out of their way to look after me. Joyously at the time, Nikki would sneak me the odd packet of Haribos. Steve, meanwhile, would go the other way. He'd be hard on me in a school atmosphere so there could be no accusations of favouritism. There I'd be in my little red dressing gown crying, but he felt it was necessary to keep that distance. At Maidwell, pupils were given demerits, a mark against their name, if they misbehaved. I had two demerits at Maidwell and they were both from Steve. They weren't for doing anything particularly bad – he just thought I needed putting back in my place. There was the occasional lighter moment, though, like the time Steve and my English teacher grabbed me by the arms and legs, and threw me, in full uniform, pens in the pocket and everything, in the swimming pool.

Steve wouldn't tolerate any nonsense when it came to cricket. We had one game where Jonny Bairstow was on the visiting team. Steve gave me out lbw and then Jonny, who'd already scored 60, bowled us out. I wasn't happy about the lbw and went round the school telling everyone Steve had made a mistake. He came down on me hard for that one. He also kept me grounded and made sure I stayed focused. He wanted me to see that success at Maidwell wasn't the be all and end all – that I knew there were bigger targets.

Cricket was far from everything. Football was still a possibility. Leicester City came knocking but they wanted me to train three nights a week. My parents objected – all that to-ing and fro-ing defeated the object of me going to boarding school. Cricket fitted in a lot better. For Leicestershire I played for their U-10s, 11s, and 12s, but they were happier to see me once a term and then leave it to the holidays.

However, whereas in sport I was always a few years advanced, academically I wasn't quite so enthusiastic. I did what I needed to do and not a lot more. That didn't mean I'd made my mind up that I was going to be a professional sportsman – that's hardly realistic at such a young age – it was just that I so loved having sport in my life. I enjoyed the way that performance was rewarded with progression. I could set myself goals and achieve them. When I first played for Loughborough Town as a 9-year-old, there was a guy called Lee Earnshaw, and I'd always think 'I'd love to be as good as him'. Eventually, I'd be better than Lee Earnshaw and find myself another goal. Those challenges remained wherever I was in my career. It wasn't just the goal that spurred me on; it was the fear of not meeting it. I was always thinking what I needed to do, not just to consolidate my game, but improve it.

When the time came for me to leave Maidwell, Steve and Nikki were upset, but my mum was quick to reassure.

'It's not the end,' she told them.

Our relationship changed then. I'd stay at the Schofields' and they became like a second family. When they had their children, Madeline and Vaughan, they became like a little brother and sister to me. There are pictures of me holding both of them when they were babies. When I got older, I remember arriving back from a trip to South Africa really late at night, going straight upstairs, waking them up and giving them a cuddle. It's hard to say what drove that connection with the Schofields, but somehow, together we clicked. They saw something in me, and, whilst I clearly wasn't analysing it at the time, I saw something in them. It's strange to have that relationship with people who aren't your blood, who you know almost by accident, but the family meant a lot to me then and they mean a lot to me now. Nikki still cuddles me, for God's sake!

Steve became someone to whom I would always go back throughout my career. Before the World Cup in 2015, he was giving me deliveries round the wicket fast with a side-arm to replicate Mitchell Johnson. It wasn't that he would coach me as such when I got older, because I didn't need it, but he would say the right things. He would simplify everything, uncomplicate it, and make everything easy. I would always come away from Steve feeling confident. He would help me feel good about myself.

After Maidwell, I had offers from Radley, Harrow, and Uppingham, three of England's great public schools. I'll be honest – they wanted me for my sporting ability rather than my brain. In the end, I chose Shrewsbury because it was best for football, and, according to my parents, there were no girls (I felt this to be a bonus back then).

Shrewsbury was incredible – beautiful buildings with vast playing fields. The latter was where I wanted to be, not the classroom. It was there I first encountered another great mentor, the former Worcestershire bowler Paul Pridgeon, now cricket manager at the school. Between Paul and Steve Schofield, I now had two incredible coaches in my corner and I cherry-picked elements from each of them. I trained incredibly hard with them and they did everything they could to make me better. They both put in extra work with me. Sometimes I'd net for three hours non-stop with Steve, and it was tough. He'd throw cricket balls at me while I was standing on a wobble board, golf balls at my head even, to get me ducking and weaving. He properly wanted to traumatise me, because then I'd be ready for the same treatment in a game. Any suggestion that I wasn't trying as hard as I should and he'd be all over me. On one occasion he threw the bucket of cricket balls at me and walked away. Three-hour sessions? I was certainly the only one I knew doing that kind of thing. Very few kids would work that hard, that consistently. I was fortunate that I loved it. In Q&As, when young players ask for my best piece of advice, I always say, 'Just enjoy it. You'll never get good otherwise – because if you don't enjoy it you won't train as much or as hard.'

Steve also recognised the value in me being stronger. He wanted me to exploit every ounce of strength to make the most of my size. He took me to see a friend who trained bodybuilders and got me into protein shakes. That pursuit of the perfect body might be seen as vain, but ultimately it saved my life.

I made my senior debut at Shrewsbury as a 14-year-old against a Worcestershire U-17 side. At Shrewsbury, age was immaterial – if you were good enough, you played. As I walked to the middle I could tell from their faces what the opposition were thinking – 'Look how small he is!' But even at that age I was strong and powerfully built. I shouldered arms to the first ball, but the second drifted into my pads and I clubbed it behind square for six. Back in the clubhouse, our wicketkeeper Jack Brydon couldn't believe it. 'I've played for the seniors for three years,' he despaired, 'and I've never hit a six. That little bugger has just hit his second ball out the park.'

Pridge is another who says right from the start it was obvious to him that I'd play international cricket, to the extent that he rang Worcester chairman John Elliott and told him, 'I've just seen a lad today who will play for England.' He goes so far as to claim the only player I compared to in terms of talent is Graeme Hick. I'm not sure about that, but it's nice to hear.

It was while I was at Shrewsbury that I played one of my favourite knocks. I was fifteen, playing for the school against Harrow in the Lord's Taverners Trophy final at Trent Bridge. They had some really good players, such as the current Kent captain, Sam Northeast, and made 220-plus in their forty overs, which for a U-15 side to chase is massive. We lost two early wickets and seemed out of the game. Batting with Joe Leach, the current Worcestershire captain, I nudged it closer and closer until we needed 12 an over for the last four overs. I got it down to 6 off the last two balls and then smashed the penultimate delivery of the game out of Trent Bridge. My mum kept all sorts of records – scorecards, newspaper cuttings – and I look back at them with a mixture of embarrassment (the haircuts) and pride (the performances) – but for sure that is one of my most treasured moments. That day, Pridge changed from 'he'll play for England' to 'he'll captain England'. He could see that I had not only the ability, but the mindset to go with it.

When that international career came, Pridge, like Steve, remained a big part of it. I'd go back to work with him again and again. If I had a one day game coming up, I'd maybe want to do some power hitting with him, or perhaps he could take a look at my technique. I trusted Pridge; he'd guided me through a lot. He'd played twenty years of first class cricket and knew what he was talking about. More than anything, though, I went back to Pridge as a mate.

In four years at Shrewsbury, I scored more than 4,000 runs at an average of 65, but for a good while, other sports remained. When it came to rugby, I had the speed and agility to make a decent scrum half. In fact, Dad always says his best memories of me playing sport are from when I was playing rugby at Maidwell, but as my height stalled at Shrewsbury, others were getting bigger. Some of the opposition were the size of men. I was captain and kicker for Shrewsbury U-15s, playing at scrum half, when I kicked ahead and then got absolutely steamrollered by the opposition's big number 8. Straight away, I felt a pain in my shoulder. I dragged myself off the floor and tried swinging my arm around. All I could hear was the sound of grinding. I had dislocated a joint in my shoulder.

I'd picked a particularly bad time to be run over by a man mountain. This was two weeks before I was going on a Leicestershire young cricketers' tour to South Africa. It would take a fairly remarkable recovery if I was going to play any sort of meaningful part, so next day Dad drove me down to Exmoor to see a physio he knew who had treated a lot of jockeys. She assured me that every rugby player in the world had broken their collarbone at some point, and then proceeded to laser my injury and strap it down, my dad following the latter part of the process very carefully. He was accompanying me to South Africa and it would be his job to strap it every day. The first week I batted practically one-handed. After that my shoulder recovered enough for me to be the top batsman on the tour.

I loved rugby but the risks clearly were too great, and it went the same way as riding and skiing as sports that had the potential to seriously affect my progression at cricket, where I showed little sign of stalling. My year group certainly helped. There were county players from Cheshire, Shropshire, Staffordshire, Worcestershire, and all over. At the same time, we had fantastic coaches and brilliant facilities indoors and out. While I was there, an indoor cricket centre was built based on the ECB's national academy. It was phenomenal. I practically lived in there, with Pridge giving me the time whenever I wanted as I strived endlessly to learn and get better. He'd be in his office writing reports and I'd be banging on the door: 'Pridge, fancy hitting some balls? Can we get the machine out?' His generosity meant I could use the indoor cricket centre at all times. He tested me, sticking me in front of a bowling machine at 75mph-plus. He would always facilitate what I wanted to do. In the early days, I used to nick off a bit because my hands would get away from me. I wanted to practise the ball moving away, and that's what I'd get. I just wanted to play and learn from my mistakes. Pridge and Steve would push me, but they also expected me to have that desire to work hard. Fine by me.

It was at Shrewsbury that I really began to get noticed. I'd already played for Midlands' representative teams, but a call-up for the England U-15s was massive. Until then I hadn't been too conscious of being a professional cricketer – I just played the game because I loved it and was good at it. When I got that call, though, something changed. Playing for England, for your country, with all the prestige that goes with it, is amazing. Even so, while I was undoubtedly being successful, and was ultra positive, I always carried a small element of negativity, a fear of failure, to push me forward. That meant that, if and when success did come, it would feel even bigger. It was the same with selection. I'd try to keep my feet on the ground by telling myself I was going to miss out. That way it would feel like a real boost when it happened, although inside I always thought I should be on the team sheet.

My parents too were good at giving me perspective. I might have played the innings of my life, and be expecting showers of praise and compliments, and all I'd get was, 'You played well there'. That was it – and I think that's a really good thing. I'm not saying it didn't irritate me sometimes, but as a sportsperson it hardens you up, and I'm a big believer that for a kid to make it, they've got to be tough. Make kids hard at a young age and they'll go a long way. My mum and dad might have praised me behind my back – I know they're super-proud – but they'd rarely do it to my face. As long as I could see that inside they were proud, I didn't mind them not pumping me up too much. Their personal and emotional investment in my career was apparent simply from the amount of time they put into it. Every Sunday they did a 300-mile round trip, from Burrough on the Hill to Shrewsbury, and then on to Evesham for me to take part in academy nets with Worcestershire. A lot of parents might not have been able to afford that, and I never took it for granted. Regardless of the money, though, they sacrificed an awful lot for me.

I was made captain of cricket at Shrewsbury. It meant a lot as it was confirmation I was the best player in the school. That's how the captaincy worked; it wasn't necessarily dished out to the person best able to lead. That's not to say I didn't have leadership qualities. An expanding cricket brain and tactical nous were carved into my character from playing so much sport with so many different people. But I wasn't mega-verbal, and I would never give an inspirational team talk. Instead, I led by example. There are many different ways of leading and that was mine. At the same time, my performances for Shrewsbury, as well as with England age group teams, were getting me noticed in the local and national sporting press, and I liked that. I enjoyed the attention. I enjoyed being the best. I loved the pressure of being the best player in the team, the one expected to do well. I far preferred to be the best than be the nobody.

Sport wasn't everything in my life. I made some great friends at Shrewsbury – and then, from the age of fifteen, there was the drinking. That was when the partying started, and for a while it never stopped. Me and my mate used to get a crate of twenty-four cans from the off licence – he had a beard and so looked older than he was, other times I'd have a fake ID – then we'd carry our purchases to the chip shop, have something to eat while hiding our drink under our chairs, and head back to school, splitting the cans between two rucksacks on the way. Then we'd head up through the schoolhouse, through a trapdoor, and on to the roof. We'd chill together, talk absolute rubbish, and have about eight cans each, after which we headed to the school bar, Tudor Court. It was all quite official – pupils had to be signed in – but we were allowed two beers, supervised, from the age of seventeen, and girls were free to go as well. If people thought we were a bit drunk, we would claim it was the beers in the bar that had got us that way.

We would drink a lot, consistently. Any time we had a spare afternoon, we'd go into pubs in town. They say there are 365 pubs in Shrewsbury, one for every day of the year, which made it slightly annoying for those pupils who got caught by teachers out on pub busts. While we were allowed to go into town, clearly the idea wasn't that we'd sit in the pub all day. But there was quite a big drinking culture among the older lads, and I liked it because it was a release – from school, from work, even from the intensity of sport. It also made me feel more confident, especially when it came to speaking to girls.

It was around about this time that my footballing dreams ended. I was playing against the Old Salopians, men who were considerably bigger than me, when I got challenged from behind, hyper-extended my foot, and damaged the ligaments in my ankle. Those weeks of recovery were the only time in my life that I didn't play any sport. It was a good excuse to drink more, but then when I was drunk I'd roll my ankle and end up making it worse. An injury that should have taken just a few weeks from which to recover ended up taking six to eight, because of me being stupid.

At night, I used to sneak out and go 'proper out' – 'out out'. That was slightly trickier. If you left the school you had to sign out and have a good excuse. The time that really got me in trouble was when I was seventeen. My best mate and I said we were going to stay with a friend's uncle and signed out on that basis. Of course, there was no uncle. We went out early and drank all day, a session that continued late into the night. If I drank a lot I'd lose my memory. I'd often have a big chunk of the evening where I didn't know what had happened. The last thing I can remember on this particular occasion is drinking champagne in a club about eleven o'clock. Next thing I knew it was 6.00 am – and I was in a hospital bed. Surprise doesn't quite describe it.

'Shit! What's happened here?'

The nurses told me I'd been found passed out on the street and an ambulance had picked me up. I had only one thought: the big trouble I'd be in if news got back to school about what had happened.

'Can I leave?'

'No.'

'But I want to go.'

'Afraid not. Until you've got somebody over eighteen to sign for you, or a member of staff from the school, you'll have to stay here.'

'What are the consequences if I leave?'

'We'll have to ring the police.'

Thinking rationally, although I was still pissed from the night before, that didn't seem likely. So I just ran out. It was about 2 miles back to school and I didn't even know the way. I was haring round roundabouts looking for signs for the right direction. Eventually, I made it back and, totally panicking, knocked on the matron's door. She was the one who looked after us all – the mother figure – and I felt I knew her well enough to confide in her. I told her what had happened and then went to bed for an hour. Ideally, I'd have slept it off but couldn't because my mum was coming to pick me up for nets at the Worcestershire Academy. We set off at eleven and I was feeling as rough as I've ever been. On the way we stopped at a café, but before the food arrived I ran out to the car park and vomited everywhere.

'You've just been sick, haven't you?' she asked when I sloped back in.

I told her I'd been out the night before, but left out the hospital side of the story.

At Worcester, I somehow managed to drag myself through the whole three-hour training session and was heading back to Shrewsbury when I had a call from my housemaster.

'You were out last night, weren't you?'

He'd picked up his phone messages and there was one from the hospital. They had obviously seen some ID on me when I'd come in and knew I was from Shrewsbury School.

'I'm sorry, James,' he continued, 'you're going to be suspended. You'll have to spend a week at home.'

My parents obviously weren't happy, but worse than that was the reaction of Pridge. He said he'd never coach me again. He felt totally let down. Pridge is a man who sticks to his word, to the extent that my parents' view was that if he wasn't going to coach me I would have to move schools. We looked at moving from Shrewsbury to Oakham, but it couldn't happen overnight, and in the meantime I went back to school. I used that time to grovel and apologise like I never had before and eventually, after a couple of weeks, Pridge backed down, but he still laid it on the line, emphasising that if I went the wrong way now it would be career threatening, and reminding me that, were I to make it as a first class cricketer I'd be under a tremendous amount of scrutiny. Pridge had seen lots of players who could have been great players cock it up. He wasn't going to let me do that. He wanted me to know I'd let him down. He'd gone out of his way to help me and I'd not given him that respect back. He'd smoothed the way for me to get in at Worcester, he'd taken me to academy training, he'd invested a lot in me. For me, my real punishment was knowing how much I'd betrayed him, how I'd lost his respect and that of the other coaches. They knew I wasn't your trademark goody two shoes. They knew I drank a lot and went out. But this was too much.

Steve was also aware that I was burning the candle at both ends. I'd come down from Shrewsbury for a net session at Maidwell and Nikki would say, 'You're smelling of booze.' She kept it from Steve but he found out about my nocturnal habits through parents of other kids at Maidwell who knew my mum and dad. To Steve it felt like I was wasting my talent. For a while he also stopped speaking to me. Like Pridge, he wanted to teach me a lesson that talent can disappear. He thought I was wasting what I'd got and what I'd developed. The blonde highlights probably didn't help. At least he didn't know about the little earring I'd had put in the top of one ear at Shrewsbury, hidden under my hair, as they weren't allowed. Nikki, though, was straight on to it: 'I know what you've done.'

'Does Steve know?' I panicked. I didn't take the risk and took it out pretty sharpish.

Not long afterwards, Steve began the silent treatment – the hate/hate times as we now call them. I went down to Maidwell to watch a game. I was walking round the boundary one way and Steve the other. Circles are tricky when you're trying to avoid someone and we ended up having a chat, albeit a frosty one. Soon after, I had a game for Shrewsbury and Steve came along to watch. Again, he was annoyed. He felt I was out of synch, a different batter, someone living off what I'd achieved rather than driving on. He rang Nikki.

'He's not the same,' he said.

The drive home to Maidwell was tense. 'I don't think your trigger is quite where it needs to be,' Steve told me.

'That's winter work,' I replied. This was June.

He flicked the indicator, pulled into a lay-by, and really let me have it. And he was right. Compared to a year previously, I had drifted. Later that year, I lived with the Schofields and got my priorities, and game, in order. I'd be in the gym at 5.30 am, have some breakfast, go for a run with Nikki, net with Steve, and then get on the weights. I was getting stronger all the time. Steve challenged me to hit a thousand balls a week. No problem – we were actually hitting 800 balls a session. It fitted Steve's mantra of 'Repeat! Repeat! Repeat!' When kids would ask me how I got so good, I'd say 'Practice – practise all the time.'

I was Steve's flagship. He saw something in me, and ultimately coached me from the age of eight to twenty-six, when I finished. He put hundreds of hours into me and never took a penny in return. He knew right from the age of nine that I was going to play for England. So when I got to fifteen and was going through that stage that all boys go through, he wasn't having it. To him it felt I was putting everything we'd invested in – and that included his family, because they were all part of the package – on the line. He felt I was betraying both my ability and them. He put me on a choker. Moving in with them kept me in line. If I'd carried on like that with the booze, there's a chance I'd be looking back on my best sporting days as being at twelve or thirteen.

I had no desire to waste my talent any more than I had to be seen as someone who wasted his talent. It reminded me horribly of how, when I first came to the school, a tutor had felt the need to have a word with me. Right from the start, I was playing cricket alongside top year pupils aged eighteen, which was unheard of. Because of that, lots of lads were jealous of me. Thing is, prior to Shrewsbury, because boys have come from a little prep school with a hundred pupils, fifteen in their class, they are used to being the best. When that is taken away, there can be an element of resentment. I would get hammered by some pupils.

'A word of warning,' my tutor told me. 'A few people are saying you're a bit arrogant.'

Oh my God! The A-word. It felt like the worst possible insult. It troubled me – I didn't want anyone to think of me like that. I didn't think I was arrogant. I felt confidence had been mistaken for something else. There is, after all, certainly in sport, a fine line between confidence and arrogance.

Whatever; it certainly got my attention. It made me have a lot more self-awareness. I didn't want anyone thinking I was arrogant any more than I would want Pridge to think I was some drunken waster who didn't care about his coaches or his talent.

Over time I became more disciplined. I still irritated Steve, though. I'd nick the remote control and make him watch *Hollyoaks* and *Home and Away*. Luckily for him, I was given a tutor flat – I'd help out round the school, coaching rugby, and be out of his hair.

That's not to say I became a monk. In the final year at Shrewsbury, everyone has their own bedsit. I had a great room, with a fire door that led on to an exterior staircase. It appeared the perfect escape route for an illicit night out, except there was a catch. The fire door was alarmed so the housemaster would know if it was opened. Early on I worked out that if I placed a magnet on the door it negated the detector. The door always appeared closed, which meant I could come and go as I pleased. Well nearly – the housemaster used to come round and check that we were in bed. My solution? I'd get a third former to sleep in mine, so when the housemaster opened the door he'd think I was there.

My mate Jonny Griffiths and I would go out twice a week until 3.00 am. Friday nights became a bit of a superstition – if there was a cricket match on the Saturday, I loved the feeling of going out to bat while a little spaced out from the night before. It was just the best time – two naughty schoolboys going out on the town, doing what we wanted, drinking WKDs, and then doing a few lessons the following morning before playing cricket. One time, though, about two weeks before the England U-19 World Cup, we got caught. At 3.00 am, just as we were just leaving a nightclub, I looked up and saw a teacher looking straight back at me.

'Taylor!' he greeted me. 'My office, 9.00 am tomorrow morning!' It was a good ten to fifteen-minute walk to school, and as I plodded back I was sure I was going to get suspended for a week. Next day, we went down to see the teacher. 'Look lads,' he said, 'I can't let this go. I'm going to have to tell somebody, which means suspension.'

I was grovelling. Proper grovelling. I'd moved up the England age groups all the way through school and with this latest discrepancy I could see my spot in England U-19s slipping away. The U-19s World Cup was imminent and no way would the management tolerate me being suspended from school after that kind of behaviour.

'I won't be able to go,' I pleaded. 'You can't tell anyone.' The conversation kept going backwards and forwards, with Jonny hiding behind me.

'Have you told anybody?' the teacher asked.

'No. No one.'

There was a pause. 'Ok,' he considered, 'I'll let this slide, but don't do it again. I haven't seen you – this didn't happen.' It was something I'd become used to – my cricket allowed me to get away with a little bit more. When it came to that U–19s World Cup, for instance, I missed two months of my A level year. The school could easily have not let me, but sportswise, they let me come and go as I pleased. I even did one of my A levels in Sri Lanka to fit in with the World Cup schedule.

Like any young lad, I wanted some fun. But, while I may have lost a little focus for a while, I was always aware there were limits. There were some loose kids at school, lads with money who wanted to make the most of it. They'd take it beyond alcohol and into drugs. I can't say the temptation was never there but I was never in the smoking and drugs gang. I had too many people to let down. My most extravagant expense at school was my haircut! I was naughty at school, but just about within the boundaries of what was acceptable, and I never let that side of me show at the various cricket centres I was involved in. They would have thought I was just a normal lad who kept his head down and never did anything.

By doing the bare minimum I needed, I still got my A levels. OK, photography might not be up there with physics or maths, but it still counts! Whatever the qualifications, it didn't matter – I lived for sport. In fact, if it had been left up to me I might well have left school when I was sixteen to pursue my future in cricket, but Mum and Dad insisted I stay and do my A levels. They would have liked me to have achieved more academically. They wanted me to have an education to fall back on if need be. While supporting me, they were always keen to emphasise that sport was unpredictable. My career could be ended at any time by an unexpected turn of events. They weren't the only ones. Before I was admitted to the Worcestershire Academy, I had an interview with its director, Damian D'Oliveira. He also emphasised that school was a very important part of my life.

'You've got to get your schooling behind you,' he told me. 'You might walk out of here, down those steps, trip up, break your leg, and that's the end of your cricketing career.' He wasn't far off right. Now people are hearing me on the radio, Dad thinks the schooling he and Mum paid for is coming up trumps. But the sport didn't turn out too badly either. There's a big poster of me in the cricket school at Shrewsbury!

Even after playing for England, I still consider school the best time of my life. No question about it, Maidwell and Shrewsbury set me up forever, and I recognise how privileged I was to go to those places. The freedom to play sport every day was amazing, while the teachers always encouraged me to push myself. I'm still in touch with a lot of friends I made there. Many of them came to our wedding. Sadly, my best mate wasn't one of them. Alex Wilson was the perfect bloke, unbelievably clever, head of house, deputy head of school, strong, good looking. He had everything to look forward to. After Shrewsbury, he went to St Andrews University. He was taking a short cut to a beach party one night when he fell from a cliff. He was nineteen. I was at an England Lions training camp when I received a phone call from a friend. 'He's gone! He's gone! Alex has gone!' I couldn't believe what I was hearing. It was awful. He meant so, so much to me – every sport, rugby, football, cricket, he was there alongside me. It hurt even more that I missed his funeral, attended by more than a thousand people, because I was on tour in South Africa. All I could be thankful for was that he and I had enjoyed a hilarious chat on Facetime just two days before he died.

I tried to block Alex's death out – cricket kept me busy – but after South Africa we went to Dubai. By now it was three months after Alex died. I was in a taxi at 4.00 am and I just broke down. I was bawling my eyes out. I rang Jose and just cried and cried. This amazing bloke, the nicest guy in the world, this lovely, lovely person – gone.

When I think of Alex I realise how lucky I am.

Chapter 3

Side Room B

It wasn't the best night's sleep I'd ever had. All the time I was hooked up to a machine monitoring my heart rate. If it went above a certain level it would alarm, if it went below a certain level it would alarm. Fine; if anything went wrong, the professionals would know right away. Thing was, these were machines calibrated for older people, not a professional sportsman in his mid-twenties. They were set so that if a heart rate dipped below sixty beats a minute, they would go off. Bearing in mind that not only was I a super-fit cricketer but I was also on drugs to lower my heart rate, I was pretty much permanently below sixty. In fact, I was getting down as low as thirty-two. No sooner had I dropped off to sleep than the machine would go mad, releasing a great shriek of a siren. The staff had never encountered this scenario before and would try to recalibrate the settings, but ten minutes later it would go off again.

It wasn't just the noise. I'm useless if there are any distractions in a room while I'm trying to sleep – the little red light on a TV, even. It has to be pitch-black and it has to be silent. Hospitals don't exactly fit that bill. It was lights everywhere, machines, chatter, people running around. The only reason I got any sleep was that, after 'running' all those marathons, my body was desperate for rest. If it hadn't been for the distractions, I could have slept on a clothes line. Jose hadn't managed much better. The nurses had to keep stepping over her to reach the machines when they went off.

As we came blurrily to life in side room B, we were still in a state of shock. By rights I should have been in a comfortable hotel bed in Cambridge and Jose should have been waking up at her family home in Shropshire. Instead, the morning light seeping through the window revealed me flat on my back, pin-cushioned with wires, and Jose in a crumpled heap on the floor. They say no two days are ever the same, and this was the living embodiment of it.

The whole horrible situation had come out of nowhere, as if someone had dealt us a brand new hand of cards – 'Here you are – sort it out!' Jose climbed on to the bed alongside me. All we could do was sit there trying to take in what had happened, to make sense of it. It was me and Jose; together we work out everything. But when it came to this particular puzzle, we didn't have a clue.

All we could do was ponder the same few questions.

'What's happened? What do we do? What does all this mean?'

There was a complete unknown of what the day was going to bring. Bemusement mixed with fear mixed with hope mixed with dread. Somewhere within all that was the vague hope that this could all be something and nothing, and normal life would resume any minute. It was a strange feeling of detachment, almost sitting back and watching your own life, waiting for something to happen. One thing we were certain about was that we wouldn't set off down the path of self-diagnosis. We decided from day one we would never Google anything to do with my condition – and that stands even now. The only result of searching for possible conditions online was catastrophising. We made a pact – 'Just don't'.

A lot of that day was about sitting there putting on a brave face. If we thought quick answers were going to come spewing forth, we were sadly mistaken. This wasn't meant to happen to me and the fact it had was going to need no small measure of investigation. All they could say at this stage was that what had occurred was probably caused by a virus, with a chance there might be a structural problem with my heart.

The consultant who looked after us that first week, Tim Robinson, was a proper cricket badger. He'd been out to follow England on their victorious Ashes tour of 2010/11 and stood alongside the Barmy Army. When he heard that 'James Taylor, the cricketer' had been brought to the cardiac unit, he had performed the medical version of a double take. Why would James Taylor, who he'd just watched on TV have the tour of his life in South Africa, have presented himself at hospital complaining of major heart issues? He told me I'd need to stay in hospital for as long as it took for more tests to be carried out.

Needles and questions. Questions and needles.

'Have there ever been any heart problems in your family?'

'No.'

'Any symptoms before?'

'No.'

Geoffrey Boycott talks about the corridor of uncertainty – I was living in it. Every search for a definitive answer seemed to lead up a blind alley.

A possible hint as to what had happened came from the fact that tests showed I'd been suffering from a virus in South Africa, as well as feeling unwell – sickness and diarrhoea – back home. In young people, the chances of a heart disorder are relatively low. A virus, I was told, might have triggered an acute form of myocarditis, an inflammation of the heart muscle that disturbs the rhythm of the heart itself. It was by some distance the preferred option – a patient can recover from myocarditis. They could live a normal life without any surgical intervention.

Tests also showed that I had glandular fever, and probably had done so for quite some time, certainly right through the tour to South Africa, possibly longer. It's an illness that makes people feel incredibly drained, so give it to someone who trains at a million miles an hour and it's going to have an impact. At the same time, I was being incredibly strict with my diet. I enjoyed being so ripped, with so little body fat, but in fact that lack of fat was putting my immune system under strain.

All the time I'd be thinking about whether I'd ever experienced anything odd with my heart before. I remembered that, occasionally, after a night out, I would say to Jose that my heart was doing funny things, I suppose mild palpitations. But I just put it down to the drinks, especially if I'd had Red Bull as a mixer. I can see that putting caffeine and alcohol in your system is not a good idea. One's a stimulant, the other's a depressant, and they're having their own little battle right there inside your body. Other than that, though, I'd never felt anything that seemed unusual or sinister.

Prior to the attack, I'd had a couple of big nights out with friends. In fact, afterwards they were worried that they might have played a big part in what happened. One had been a night in Nottingham with a few mates. My drinks of choice were usually beer or vodka, lime and soda. I generally refused to do jager bombs because I knew I wouldn't be able to sleep afterwards because of the caffeine in the Red Bull, but that night the alcohol I'd already had made me waver and I did about ten – and that's a lot for a little guy. You can tell the state I was in because Jose was in the club we ended up in and I left without even saying goodbye to anyone, including her.

Another time, I went to watch the rugby in Wales. It was a 9.00 am start in Shrewsbury. We had a crate of bottled beer, another crate of cans, and then champagne as well. We watched Wales v Italy in Cardiff, had more drinks afterwards around the town, and then headed back to Shrewsbury for more drinking until 4.00 am. These were sizeable sessions, but then again, I'd been having blowouts all my life, just like plenty of others my age. There was nothing to suggest that these were anything different. I was just letting my hair down, living my life.

Instead of the fleeting affair I was hoping for, the machine by my bed became my constant companion. It analysed my heart's performance 24/7 and at first was exceptionally scary. I couldn't help but watch the lines, so when one of these worms would occasionally go haywire it would inevitably send my anxiety through the roof – I think that's what they call a vicious circle. There was plenty enough anxiety going on as it was without this machine behind me reminding me of my mortality and vulnerability every second. It played on my mind all the time.

Those first few days were an endless series of tests and scans. My lack of movement, meanwhile, meant the doctors had to thin my blood once or twice a day. It was like being punctured as they stuck the needle in the little fat roll at the bottom of my stomach.

Anyone who has found themselves suddenly in hospital will tell you how they long for normality. Nothing spectacular – how you just wish you could be yourself. I couldn't have that, but I had Jose.

When it was clear I wouldn't be going home, she immediately made the decision to stay with me, however long it took. She moved up from off the floor on to the comparable luxury of a camp bed. Not that sleeping was any easier. For the next two nights, the constant alarming continued, before the machine eventually realised, with a little help from the nurses, I was in my mid-twenties, not my seventies. Frustrating as it was, staying in hospital made sense. Usually, just lying there would have driven me mad, but there was nowhere I wanted to be more. I was physically drained, ashen, exhausted. I couldn't walk because my body was so wrecked from what it had been through. The only place I ever went was the few feet to the loo. I didn't shower for three days because I couldn't be without the monitor on – I didn't want to be without the monitor on! And when you think about how badly I sweated on that first day, that really is quite something. I'm surprised anyone came near me. But I just wasn't interested, and neither was Jose. There was only one thing we were thinking about – my heart and where it would lead us.

As the days passed, I began to sleep better in hospital, to the extent I was sleeping better than I had been at home. I'd begun to realise whatever was going to happen on that unit was out of my control, so, in a weird sort of way, there was less to worry about in there than in normal life on the outside. I think my body was still coming to terms with the intense stress it had been under too.

However, it never got easier waking up in hospital. Every single morning the same horrible realisation would slowly sink in – 'Oh God – we're here!'

All that time, while the uncertainty over my condition was unsettling, I was trying to remain positive. On the third day, I put on Instagram 'What doesn't kill you makes you stronger'. It was a cartoon of a mouse lifting itself free of a trap. I wasn't to know then that my condition offered no such escape.

All the time, I was trying to keep my situation quiet. My phone was going mad with people trying to find out what was going on. It was like that for the first week, but I was determined that only close people should know. I've always been good at blocking things out and hiding things. It's part of being a professional cricketer – very few players, for instance, are totally honest about injuries – and this was no different. I didn't want there to be a lot of external chatter about me being in hospital. That kind of thing can be damaging. It can leave a lasting impression and could have affected my selection for England. The result was that for a whole week barely anyone knew I was in hospital. My teammates and my family did, but no one else. I didn't even tell some of my friends. If people texted me, I'd tell them I wasn't very well – I had a bad cold. It wasn't like I could give an explanation if I wanted to. I had no idea what was going on any more than anybody else, so what was I meant to say? I was just hoping that I was going to be all right. Those who I did tell were totally gutted for me when I said it was an issue with my heart. My friend and former Nottinghamshire teammate Sam Wood (Woody) initially thought my hamstring had gone. When he discovered it was my heart, he couldn't believe what he was hearing. My sister also rang. My parents wanted to hide it from her until they knew exactly what was happening, but they were worried she might hear something via the media. Their worries were justified. My agent, the former Somerset, Derbyshire and Lancashire wicketkeeper Luke Sutton, was increasingly having to field enquiries from the press. Not only had I disappeared halfway through the game at Cambridge, but I'd missed the first Championship game of the season against Surrey. An England cricketer had vanished into thin air and the media understandably wanted to know why.

'What's wrong with him? Someone tell us.'

Inevitably, word slipped out that I was in hospital. Luke took all the enquiries and could only tell the truth. 'He's having tests – when there's anything to add we'll let you know.'

With the answers we wanted so far unforthcoming, we began asking family and friends, those with a link to the medical profession, if we'd be better going private. But people pointed out that if we went private we would be seeing exactly the same doctors, and these were the best in the business. I had to stay positive. The tests had shown nothing seriously untoward and we were just waiting on the results of an MRI scan, which delivers a more detailed analysis of an issue. With nothing cast iron to say otherwise, there was still a part of me thinking I could be out in time for the Sri Lanka series. Jose was also being ultra positive. She kept telling me to look at it like having a broken leg. 'These things happen,' she'd say, and after a recovery I'd be back. Even if it turned out to be a longer term lay-off, I was thinking, 'OK, if that's what it takes, I'll have it.'

I was attached to the machine for the first five days. Then I was given an ambulatory monitor, a portable pack that allowed me more independence. It made me feel a little better; it was a step forward, even if only to hobble to the water fountain to fill up my juice bottle.

On day six, however, everything changed. Jose and I were sitting on the bed doing word searches on my iPad. Sounds a bit sad, I know, but we were actually really enjoying it! I was having a really good time. Mum was there too. Then we heard the swish of the curtains. It was Tim. We'd got to know him well during the week. When he'd delivered other news or results, he'd breezed in, 'Hi James. All looks good.' This time he was different, much more tentative. He came in, got a chair, and sat down. That didn't bode well. Jose got off the bed and sat down too.

'The boys are doing well,' said Tim – small talk referring to Nottinghamshire's latest match. It was meant to break the ice, but instead seemed really ominous. Let's face it; everyone in that room knew he hadn't come to talk about the cricket. I was thinking, 'Don't beat around the bloody bush'. He paused, and then he just said it: 'Your scan is abnormal.'

And at that point everything just crashed.

'It's something seen in people with arrhythmogenic right ventricular cardiomyopathy,' he continued. Just those words – those horrible ugly words. I couldn't take it in.

'Fuck off. Fuck off, mate. Fuck off. Fuck off.' I wasn't being aggressive. I just couldn't absorb what he was saying. Jose got up and climbed on the bed with me.

'No exercise,' he continued. 'No cricket. It's genetic. If you have children, they might get it.'

My heart just dropped. It was an awful, awful feeling, like someone had shot me in the stomach.

Tim pulled a device from his pocket, wires trailing from it. 'You're going to need this – it's a defib.' It was like a ton of bricks falling on us at once.

There was a moment of trying not to cry, battling back the tears. But it was too hard. As soon as I started I couldn't stop. Up to that point, all the way through hospital I'd done my utmost to keep it together, trying my hardest not to cry. But there's only so long you can keep that up, and then when it comes out, it really comes out. The tears flowed.

Jose was hugging me, cradling me. 'It can't be. It can't be,' I just kept saying it over and over again.

My mum was speechless. She was tapping her leg. Over and over, tapping her leg. None of us had prepared for this. In our heads, at worst we were preparing for them to come in and say, 'This is a viral problem. You're going to be out of cricket for a while but it can be sorted.' I'd even come round to the possibility of having six months off. But then, in a single moment, all that had gone. All that hope, that investment in thinking I still had a chance, gone. Everything. Gone.

We were numb. Tim followed it up with the medical explanation of what had happened, but it wasn't registering. I couldn't take it in. It was just a voice.

'What about drinking?'

Looking back, it sounds an odd thing to ask, but at that point I was subconsciously clawing at anything. My brain just needed to hear something that wasn't about loss – that a semblance of normality could remain.

'Well, you can have the odd beer,' he said. It didn't matter. I couldn't have cared less. My brain had just been buried by an avalanche. In that suffocating darkness it was thrashing around searching for the tiniest glimmer of light.

In the end, there was only one thing able to penetrate the utter despair of that moment. 'If it's any consolation,' said Tim, 'in 80 per cent of people this condition is found in post-mortem.' In my shoes, that day in Cambridge, four out of five people would have been dead. That's the fact of the matter. I was the other one.

Clearly having no idea at the scene unfolding down the corridor, Steve Schofield, the man who'd taught me so much, had arrived to visit. His whole family were outside. I was adamant: 'They can't come in.' Jose went out to see them. She thought I needed a few minutes alone with my mum. There's no one stronger than Mum in a crisis – lose her phone and she's in a flap, but when it's something serious, there's no one better. She was exactly the same here. She'd basically just heard that her son's life was over as he knew it, but she was calm personified. I didn't see her cry. We're not that sort of family. 'I'm just glad you're still here,' she told me. But inside I could tell she was devastated. Dad arrived soon after and he showed exactly the same strength. Together they did what they could, in circumstances where no one could do anything.

I changed my mind about the Schofields. 'It's not going to make a difference is it? If they're here they might as well come in. We might as well face it together.'

When they realised what had happened, they were in hysterics as well. Steve had wanted to be a professional cricketer but hadn't made it. Having coached me from such a young age, he'd invested so much of himself in me. I crumpled in his arms. 'We'll do it again,' he cried. 'We'll do it all again.'

I wanted to see Vaughan and Madeline. I tried really hard to keep it together as I cuddled them.

I'd always looked at my life as a series of chapters. Something would happen and then I'd box it off. Maybe some people would say that's not particularly healthy, that I shouldn't parcel up episodes of existence and stack them away, but equally I found it helpful to always look forward, not back. If ever I needed to look forward, now was the time.

I knew that I couldn't let this destroy me. When it came to me and Jose especially, we could either let this beat us up or we could make the best of a bad situation.

Within an hour of being told the news, my view was clear. 'I'm retiring. Done.' The way I looked at it, I'd got a big enough battle on my hands without some long torturous debate over whether I should wait for another diagnosis, a glimmer of hope. As much as the retirement, I also just wanted people to know where I was, where I was at. I'd been in a hospital for a week, vanished from real life. Barely anybody knew what it was all about.

'This has happened,' I said. 'Let's just get it out there and move on.' I'm always about moving forward and this was no different. I knew from my batting that if I didn't tell people there was a problem it would make it incredibly hard to deal with. It all builds up in your head. You're fighting enough as it is without fighting with yourself. That's a tough place to be.

My mind was clear. 'My life as I know it is done. Let's crack on. What's next?'

I rang Luke that day: 'Let's get on with it.' He was devastated just like everyone else, but equally he knew exactly what I was like. At no point did he try to talk me out of it. He understood how my mind worked. For me, as a human being, he knew what was needed.

When everyone had gone, and it was back to me and Jose, we lay on the bed together. We were both raw with the tumult of the day, the sheer torrent of emotion. The tears came again for both of us. But at the same time something had changed. We both understood that to survive we had to face up to a new us, a new reality. We had reached the same conclusion: 'We can either carry on crying or we can make the best out of a horrible situation.'

It had been another long and bruising day, one that had ripped both of us up inside. Eventually, I fell into an exhausted but restless sleep. In the middle of the night, I woke. As I opened my eyes, just for the briefest moment I thought the events of the day before had been a dream. It was all OK. I was going to be all right. I could carry on playing cricket and everything would be fine. And then the reality came crashing back in. I recalled everything that I'd been told. 'No more cricket. No more exercise. Your children might get it.'

I just screamed.

'Oh no!'

It was the worst thing. Jose got off the camp bed and comforted me as I wept.

Chapter 4

Ambition

Having been Worcestershire Academy player of the year two years on the trot, and with the club itself for four years, many would have assumed that when it came to me progressing into first class cricket they would be top of the list.

But after success all the way through school, club cricket, and regional and national age groups, I was fortunate that Worcestershire was not the only county interested in taking me on. Warwickshire had first talked to me about a contract when I was sixteen. I played in a second team game for Worcestershire against them and got back to back 50s. Their second XI coach Keith Piper pulled me aside and asked me if I'd be interested in joining. It was all very unofficial and, to be honest, at sixteen, I didn't even know what a contract was, so it all petered out into nothing.

In the end, Leicestershire beat Worcestershire to it in terms of actually offering me a contract. They knew I was a local lad and had seen me play with England U-19s. Worcestershire got very agitated when they found out and offered me terms too. Warwickshire also came back into the running, but in the end it wasn't a hard decision – I was a Leicestershire boy after all. Not only that, there were opportunities to get in the Leicestershire side that just weren't there at Worcestershire. At New Road, I was competing with the likes of Graeme Hick, Ben Smith, Vikram Solanki, and Phil Jaques. In the second team were Moeen Ali and Daryl Mitchell. They were all ahead of me in the pecking order. I was going to struggle to get in the first team.

I was still at school when I had a secret meeting with the Leicestershire coach Tim Boon and chairman in a pub in Loughborough. We agreed a deal. Their offer was the lowest of everyone, but they offered me something their competitors couldn't – progression. It was a brave decision to move counties at that age, and it's not a common occurrence. It would have been so much simpler to stay put at Worcestershire where I knew everyone. But it's easy to stay in your comfort zone; throughout my career I would always take the path that allowed me to improve. I've always been good with change – good job, as it's turned out. You have to make the most of whatever is put in front of you. For me it was a straightforward decision to go to Leicestershire, but I had no idea if it was going to work.

When I told Worcestershire I was going to Leicestershire, it went down like the proverbial shit sandwich. Understandable – they'd invested a lot of money, time and effort in me. But equally they hadn't acted on making the association permanent until someone else had come along. Leicestershire had made the positive move and Worcestershire were just reacting. Their director of cricket, Steve Rhodes, went over to see my mum and dad in an attempt to persuade me to stay. But Tim had already done his talking. My dad in particular thought Leicestershire the better option, and I was inclined to agree. It felt like they saw my potential better than Worcestershire, and the fact I had a history with the club was another clincher. I knew a lot of the lads at Leicestershire – Josh Cobb and Nathan Buck were just two of those I had played with through the age groups at the county – and it was easier to slot in from that point of view. I didn't know many of the senior lads, but there weren't too many egos knocking round, and the dressing room felt welcoming.

Leicestershire isn't a big club but it would be top of the league for approachability and friendliness. Tim, in particular, was great. He was very positive, lively and energetic, and had plenty of time for me. I loved batting and that appealed to him. He took me under his wing and over the next four years turned me from a good school cricketer into someone ready for the international stage. Tim was quite a technical coach but he always kept it simple for me. I never liked to overcomplicate and he knew what got me going from quite early on. His time, effort, patience and expertise were just what I needed as he taught me the fundamentals of first class batting. I began to understand what my downfalls were.

My progression at Leicestershire was as quick as I'd hoped. Essentially, I leapt straight from school cricket into first class cricket, probably before I was ready, but Tim took that chance on me. At that point I wasn't necessarily the best batsman in the Leicestershire team, but I made my claim for a place stronger by virtue of my fielding. It was a great example of me finding a way to get into a team, giving myself a unique selling point that people couldn't ignore. It was more subconscious than that, but that purpose was there nonetheless.

My first season was really tough. I only played a handful of games and made my debut when I was still at school. My first fixture? You guessed – Worcestershire at New Road. It was weird going back, especially as I'd trodden on a few toes by leaving, but later Steve Rhodes wrote me a really positive letter wishing me well. I appreciated that. I never want to burn bridges, just the same as I've tried not to burn them with anyone else. That's why it's important to have people around you who can do the more bullish stuff that I certainly didn't want to do as a 17- or 18-year-old and I don't particularly want to do now. Bullish is the last thing my heart needs me to be. When it came to dealing with the move from Worcestershire, I had my parents in that role. I wouldn't have known how to deal with it. The attitude of my parents was much more, 'If this needs to be done, then we'll be the ones who'll do it.'

Despite Tim's best attempts, there's only so much you can do in a short space of time. That first season, I was what I was – a schoolboy cricketer playing first class cricket. I didn't know my technique well enough. When I was in, I knew how to score runs, but early on, against experienced, and sometimes international bowlers, it wasn't a good combination.

But I was always wanting to learn, and getting on really well with the older lads undoubtedly helped. I had no qualms about talking to them because of the years I'd already had alongside more senior players. Paul Nixon, our veteran wicketkeeper, was amazing. The energy he had, the passion for the game, was phenomenal. Then there were the Kolpaks – overseas players, generally South African, not considered as such because of their countries' deal with the EU – H.D. Ackerman, Boeta Dippenaar, Claude Henderson. A lot of people didn't agree with Kolpaks, claiming they stopped young English players getting into the team, but they didn't stop me. The education I got from them – pacing an innings, game plans, technical advice – was invaluable. When I got my Test call-up against South Africa, Boeta rang me to say best of luck. I hadn't spoken to him for three years. 'Trust yourself,' he said. 'Go and do your thing.' It was amazing. It showed the kind of man he is.

Ackerman, meanwhile, showed me the value of resilience, wanting to bat all day, loving to score runs – and also how to be selfish. Every batsman has to be selfish to a certain extent, not wanting to let anyone else do it. Batsmen need that mindset. Ultimately, Leicestershire was where I learned to take responsibility. I wanted to be selfish, to be the person who was not out at the end, to get the job done. Ackermann might not always have done things perfectly, he might have rubbed people up the wrong way, but me being an impressionable 18-year-old, I just wanted to learn off him the whole time. I respected him for the cricketer and man he was.

In some respects, I was already ahead for my age. My game awareness, for instance, was better than most. I was a bit of an old head on young shoulders.

Patience, valuing your wicket, never wanting to give it away, aren't always virtues associated with young players. But I learnt from every opportunity I got. Even when I got it wrong I learnt from my mistakes. I was never one to think 'Oh well, no problem – I've got another innings in two days'. Right from a young age I wrote down all my scores, added them up every half season, and worked out my averages. I always wanted to score the most runs I possibly could and knew the best way of doing that was being at the crease. The best piece of advice I got from Boeta was very simple but it always stuck with me: 'You've got to make the most of every innings. When you get in, don't get out, because next time you start again on nought.' That was my big thing – 'I'm in now. I'm going nowhere.' Starting again isn't just about the score – the first thirty to fifty balls of an innings are so important because they are the hardest. After that it's a lot easier. I took that mentality through my career.

When the 2009 season came around, Tim's work on my technique over the winter paid immediate dividends. Before the end of April I made my debut first class hundred, 122 not out, helping to save the game as we followed on against Middlesex at Southgate. How I did it I'm unsure. I'd had a shocking night's sleep. I was room sharing with our spinner Carl Crowe, and he snores like anything. The feeling when I got to a hundred was one of massive relief – confirmation that I could play at this level. I hadn't done anything different to what I normally did, but I'd performed. I knew that mentally I had what it takes. Now it was just a matter of doing it on a consistent basis. Afterwards, Tim insisted we had a glass of champagne in the dressing room. It was about recognising a special achievement; having people around you who want to share your success makes such a massive difference. Soon after, I got a hundred in a one dayer against … er … Worcestershire. That gave me confidence, and confidence is massive in any sport. My plan was to progress and that's exactly what I was doing. Chances are, if I'd have stayed at Worcester I wouldn't have been among the opposition.

Other things were changing. While I was a hooligan at school in terms of going out drinking, when I got to Leicestershire I did so less and less, because I knew it was a professional environment. I wasn't going to step on anybody's toes. It was also a bit of an odd mixture – lads who were either really young or really mature – so we tended to follow the lead of the older guys. Yes, when we won a game – when we eventually won a game – we would have a blowout, but the focus was all on the cricket. That was a blessing for me because it was exactly what I needed to get better. Cricket was the absolute number one priority. If anything, I did too much. I hit too many balls. But that was just the way I operated and ultimately it shaped who I was as a cricketer, establishing a work ethic and helping me understand my game. Temptation had also been sidelined in another way. I was living at home with my parents in the middle of nowhere – going out wasn't exactly easy! I was nineteen and boring as anything.

That first full season was a big learning curve for me. One day cricket was fine, but red ball cricket was tough with the ball zipping around, delivered by better and more consistent bowlers. But I still trusted myself to do well, knowing I would find a technique that worked. I must have been doing something right because at the end of the season I was voted the Cricket Writers' Club Young Cricketer of the Year. I'd scored 1,177 first class runs in sixteen matches at an average of 58.85 with three hundreds, including my first double hundred, against Surrey at The Oval, and six 50s.

It led to a call-up for the England Lions – another target met on the road I'd mapped out for myself. Succeed at school – graduate into county cricket. Succeed at county cricket – graduate into the Lions. Succeed at the Lions – graduate into the full England side.

Targets – there were always targets: scores to beat, people to get better than. If there was a catching competition, I'd try to win it. Who's going to put their hand up and score the most? That'll be me. It was a question of ticking the box at one level and then trying to reach the next – and that's what I did.

At first on that initial Lions tour in Dubai against Pakistan, I was frustrated, carrying the drinks when I felt I should have been playing. When I did get my opportunity, I took it, scoring a couple of 50s in the one dayers in seriously tough 40 degree heat against a team with full internationals playing. It felt good showing off in front of people, some of whom might well have been doubters. Aged nineteen, having come from the second division, questions would have been asked of my ability. The runs I'd scored in county cricket would have been countered with a 'Yes, but the second division is easy', which is what I tell people now, because there is a big difference, but I knew I was good enough to compete with the players in the Lions, and it soon became apparent they saw me as competition.

Take one senior international cricketer. We had been getting on so well on that trip – for the first part at least when I was 12th man. We used to hang around together and go shopping. I respected him. Then as soon as I started playing, an edge developed between us. I was now a threat and that changed the dynamic. It was something I'd get more and more used to as a young player challenging more experienced lads. I learned you have to be careful who you surround yourself with in a cricket team. Surround yourself with insecure people and they'll put you down to make themselves feel better. I became very aware of that, so if anyone did make a comment I would know why they'd done it. Their criticism wasn't about making me feel bad; it was about giving them a boost.

Don't judge these players. Insecurities are a cricketer's constant companion. It's tough growing up trying to make a name, worrying what other people are thinking. If anything, I was hypersensitive myself, so I might have been reading meanings into situations and words a little bit too much. Hyper-awareness is as dangerous as blind arrogance. Then again, if you see someone whispering in a corner, it's hard not to wonder if they're whispering about you.

You only truly comprehend the peculiarities of dressing room psychology through age and experience. Over time you learn to understand what parts of you work around other people, and what parts they aren't willing to accept. That's why in my later years I was so confident in myself, which then helped with my cricket.

I tried not to worry too much about agendas within the team. Experiencing tour life with the Lions at such a young age was unbelievable – making friends with some of the best players in the country, staying in great hotels, seeing somewhere as amazing as Dubai. I just wanted to get better and enjoy myself. I just wanted to show what I could do. I loved it.

In the following two seasons, I cemented my place in the Leicestershire lineup, regularly scoring runs in all formats of cricket. I loved the club but knew ultimately I needed to play for a bigger outfit in the first division if I was going to fulfil my ambitions. Before I moved on, though, the Leicestershire boys delivered one truly magnificent achievement: winning the T20. Ours was a team with no egos, no star players. Instead, everybody played a role. Everybody knew what they needed to do. It's another thing to then go out and do it, but that's exactly what we did. Our template as a team was perfect. On the road to Finals Day, everybody in our dressing room won a game at some point. Someone would always put that little piece in the jigsaw. Somerset, who we played in the final, had Kieron Pollard, Jos Buttler, Marcus Trescothick, James Hildreth and Peter Trego. No one gave us a cat in hell's chance – and that made it even better. I loved that day – massive crowd, noise, excitement. It was just class. One of the best feelings ever, combined with a terrible haircut on my part.

Whilst the T20 win was an incredible moment, and Leicestershire had been great for me, I needed that new challenge. I wanted consistently to compete against better players, play at a bigger ground, train with internationals every day, and improve my standards. I wanted to be somewhere I would have to fight for a place, and I wanted to win trophies, more than the T20, in four day and one day cricket. Tim had also announced his departure, and that certainly helped seal the decision; I would no longer have this batting guru holding my hand.

There were four clubs showing an interest – Warwickshire, Lancashire, Nottinghamshire and Somerset. After winning theT20, Leicestershire went out to the Champions Trophy in India and it was there that Somerset approached me. But Taunton felt like too big a geographical move at that time in my life. It was also a batsman's paradise, and I didn't want people to say I was getting easy runs. I wanted to be tested, so when I did score runs it would matter and get me noticed.

Peter Moores, the then Lancashire coach, came to see me at home, but I wasn't sure about Lancashire. I didn't like Old Trafford as a ground. That narrowed it down to Warwickshire and Nottinghamshire. Warwickshire were the odds-on favourites. I had meetings with head coach Ashley Giles, looked around apartments, figured out where I wanted to live, and thought their offer was brilliant. I really felt wanted by them. They'd made overtures in my direction the previous year as well. At the time, I'd thought that was a year too early. Now, however, the time felt right, and Edgbaston also appealed as Jose was at university in nearby Leamington Spa.

My parents, however, always wanted me to go to Nottinghamshire, a club I'd never really considered. They liked Trent Bridge, and, thinking about it, so did I. It was, after all, where I'd played one of the most memorable shots of my career, clubbing the ball out of the ground to win that Lord's Taverners final. I had a chat with the club and they were really keen. They invited me down to have a look round and said all the things I wanted them to say. I couldn't help but be impressed. Also, this was just the sort of testing pitch I was looking for. In the end I didn't need much persuading. I already knew a few of the lads, such as Alex Hales and Luke Fletcher, and Harry Gurney moved from Leicestershire with me. Anyway, I always went with what my parents thought!

It wasn't as simple as it looked, though, and it didn't take long for things to get messy. With a year left on my contract, having originally said I could leave, Leicestershire then said they wanted money. It posed a major hurdle – it was virtually unheard of in county cricket for players to be bought out of a contract. If I was going to leave Leicester, I would be one of the first ones. I ended up having a heated conversation with the captain, Matthew Hoggard.

We were at a function and went outside to talk in his car. We were arguing, going backwards and forwards.

'You haven't earned the right to leave,' he told me.

'What? You can't be serious? I'm averaging over 50 in first class cricket and you're telling me I haven't scored the runs to deserve a move?'

Hoggy felt I should continue to learn my trade at Leicestershire. I'm not one for confrontation, but I wasn't having that. It was a load of rubbish.

'How can you possibly say that? I've been here four years and given everything for this club.'

It was very out of character for me to go back at someone like that, but if I think I'm right I will defend myself. Hoggy was a big lad, ex-England star, Ashes hero, but at that moment I thought he was out of order and so let him have it back. I can understand why Leicestershire did what they did – they were losing one of their best young batsmen – but I wanted to progress and nothing was going to get in the way of that.

In the end, Nottinghamshire made a payment to Leicestershire and the move was complete. It had been a bit of an odd way to finish at a club that meant a lot to me then, and still does. I owe a lot to Leicestershire – the way they looked after me, brought me on, backed me, and gave me opportunities. I retired at twenty-six having played well over a hundred first class games, which is unheard of, and so much of that is down to them. Thanks to Leicestershire I was two years more advanced than anyone else my age in the country.

Sadly, Leicestershire have been cast adrift in recent years. The truth is, they just don't have the money, and without it they can never be a powerful force. Are there too many counties? Try closing them down! All I know is they are a great club, with great people, but to meet my own challenges I had to move on.

Straight away at Nottinghamshire I noticed the difference. It was chalk and cheese. I couldn't believe what we had at Trent Bridge compared to what we didn't have at Grace Road – the facilities, the kit, the food, everything was a cut above. Trent Bridge being an international Test ground changed the atmosphere completely. It felt vibrant and more competitive. The sheer number of people around the place, staff and spectators alike, was startling.

Preparation at Nottinghamshire was much more professional, while being around those actually playing international cricket, as opposed to those aspiring to that level, made a big difference. The whole setup was 100 per cent more aspirational, the next stepping stone to international cricket, playing against international cricketers along the way. The games themselves were far more competitive. The pitches too were tough, not what I was used to, and instead of two good bowlers coming at me, there were three or four. It felt like I was in a battle for the whole eighty overs. In second division cricket a batsman could get through fifty overs and then cash in for the next thirty before the new ball came along. That was rarely the case in first division cricket.

The change in the dressing room also took some getting used to. I was a bit naïve coming from Leicestershire, where there tended to be more mellow characters, and also I'd grown up alongside some of the players. The banter at Trent Bridge was a little bit more full on. At that stage of my career, I was always more minded to take a back seat when I walked into a new changing room. I wasn't the sort to go in there all guns blazing. Better to review the scene and introduce myself gradually. For a while I sat back and watched before adding my voice. I'd still cop it but not quite as much. As soon as I got a little bit chirpier I certainly copped it a lot more. Alex Hales, Luke Fletcher, Paul Franks – there were some hilarious guys in the Nottinghamshire dressing room who brought banter to the next level. They could be ruthless. If you gave it, you had to expect to take it back. It was a tough education in what a high-class competitive dressing room can be like, but equally it was one that I needed. It was a necessary process. It took me a while to adjust but I needed to man up. On the pitch I was as tough as they come, but I needed to learn more about how teams operate back in the pavilion and it made me grow in that environment.

Out on the field, I found that first season at Nottinghamshire hard. I was averaging 35, which was as good as anyone else in the team, but assistant coach Wayne Noon felt he needed to have a dig. 'Is there any danger of you repaying us for the money we spent on you with some runs?' he snapped.

OK, I wasn't making the scores I wanted, but I was digging in, getting 30s off seventy or eighty balls, making runs in really tough situations, valuable contributions, which was exactly what the side needed. More often than not we were two wickets down early on and I was going in and fighting for my team. The comment shocked and astonished me. Noon knew that a 22-year-old going to a club like Nottinghamshire, a Test match ground, having been bought out of a contract, was a massive move. That was already enough pressure to live up to.

I'm a very positive person, the sort who needs an arm round the shoulder rather than someone telling me I'm a waste of space. I didn't often blow up at a coach but this was different. It was the most disrespectful thing I'd ever heard. I turned round. 'You fucking idiot.' There was an anger he had said it to me, but there was an anger also that he had said it to anybody. It's such a dumb thing for a coach trying to get the best out of a team to say to one of his players. It's your team, so treat people in a way that will help them perform.

Falling out with Noon that soon into my Nottinghamshire career was problematic. As a young player I needed someone to help me, and yet there was this tension between us from very early on. That's a tough place to be. I know as both a coach and a player that a decent progressive relationship needs respect and it didn't feel like it was there between us. I'd been in all sorts of different environments, like Leicestershire and the Lions, so I knew how things were done elsewhere. Maybe that was the issue with Noon – I wasn't his player. I was the product of other systems. He formed opinions of me that were totally wrong. Don't get me wrong; taking criticism from coaches or teammates is normal for professional sports people, but it needs to be constructive criticism, rather than just criticism.

I didn't mind people giving me stick if I'd done something wrong – fine. In fact, I don't mind any manager hammering players so long as they then pump them up as well. Criticism when things go wrong needs to be at least on an equal basis with the encouragement and praise that comes when things go right. It's the same with emotion. Show you care, but not with consistently negative emotion.

I respect Mick Newell a great deal but again there were times when we were struggling as a team when we would clash. I just felt the negativity was getting too much. I would snap. We lost at Durham and Mick called me weak in front of the rest of the lads. He was just frustrated and probably didn't mean it in the way it came across, but I just blew up. If you want to fire me up then 'weak' is the word to call me!

Sometimes I think we forget that managers also need good people around them to help form a healthy environment. I felt like Mick needed that support, and when Peter Moores was added to the coaching staff he was the man who provided it – ultra positive, a great man manager. Peter knows individuals and what makes a team tick. He knows you don't just keep players down.

At Nottinghamshire, I increasingly found myself fending for myself. Ultimately, I had higher ambitions, to play for England, and if I wasn't going to have the coaches' help, I would have to look after myself. That's an average position in which to find yourself, but I was lucky because I had that basic love of cricket, which always dragged me out of that negative environment. When Peter came in, he dragged me out of it too. Peter is all about making me, or any other player, better. He was there for half a season and in three months I never had a bad net. That doesn't mean I hit every ball perfectly. It means when that net was finished I'd taken away something from it. I averaged around 80 while Peter was at the club. Now he's a great mentor for me with my coaching. Forget all the negative stuff you've read about Peter Moores – he's a progressive thinker and an excellent coach.

At any club there will be periods where the road feels a little bumpier than you'd like, but the vast majority of my time at Nottinghamshire was a fantastic journey on a well-oiled machine geared not for survival but for success. It was a hugely enjoyable period. I'd never had so much fun playing cricket. In my second year we won the YB40 final at Lord's. It was another massive moment for me. I went to my first Lord's final when I was eleven, when Somerset beat Leicestershire in a game many remember for the Leicestershire medium pacer Scott Boswell getting the yips. Ever since that day it had always been a dream of mine to play on that same stage, so to be one of those players on the balcony celebrating, as I'd seen so many do before, was an incredible moment. One of the best feelings in sport is childhood ambitions achieved.

Next season I was offered the biggest honour the club could bestow on a player – the captaincy. At that time, being only twenty-four, I felt the four day captaincy was a step too far at too early a point in my career. I didn't honestly feel I was ready. Instead Chris Read carried on in that job while I led the one day team. But it felt special to have been asked. Nottinghamshire's was far from an inexperienced dressing room – there were a lot of very successful players who'd been there a long time – so it felt like a huge amount of trust had been put in me. I did occasionally captain the four day team when Chris was injured, but I never felt like I'd made the wrong decision turning it down full-time. It would have looked great on my CV, but I didn't feel I needed to take it all on at once. I was already living the life I'd always wanted as a cricketer. The atmosphere at every T20 game was phenomenal, the fans were so friendly and supportive, we consistently won games, and I was contributing to our success while having fun along the way. Amazing times.

However your sporting life is going – good, bad or indifferent – you need an escape, to be able to switch off. Alex Hales was a close mate of mine at Trent Bridge and in those first few years we went out a lot more than we should have done, which when you're striving for international recognition isn't exactly ideal. But then again, I'd never lived in a city, never lived on my own, so I'd never had the opportunity to go out round town and stumble back home again. I was going to enjoy life and I didn't need to look too far to find a few companions wishing to do the same. While there were players who enjoyed a drink at Leicestershire, it never compared to Nottinghamshire. This was different gravy.

I still worked hard at my cricket; I just burned the candle at both ends. Gradually that tapered down a little, but even so, I did make the odd mistake. During a rainy Championship game at Worcester, for instance, I got back late to the hotel. I had no money to pay the taxi and was hammering on the hotel door to wake someone up. I think I was still drunk on the way to the ground. I don't even remember getting there. All I recall is that, on the way to the dressing room, some of the boys put me in a big industrial dustbin. When I crawled out, I made my way up to the dressing room. Unfortunately, the fact that I was being so loud and such an idiot meant the people who'd been out with me – Hales and Samit Patel – got into trouble as well. Thankfully, we were only required to field for ten to fifteen overs at the end of the day, but then Samit, Hales and I were made to do naughty boy running, i.e. fitness training. It got worse. We had a team meal that night and because I'd got a Worcester connection I had to organise it, book it, and do a little speech. All I wanted to do was go to bed.

Hales and I were two very different characters who enjoyed going out and being lads, until eventually I just about managed to grow up!

In the season I retired, Nottinghamshire were relegated. It was tough for the club but it was also a blessing in disguise as it prompted change – a change that I'd been advocating for the previous two years. Newell moved upstairs, allowing Moores to come in as full-time coach. Sometimes you need something drastic to happen to force action.

For me, sadly, Moores' arrival was too late. Cambridge had occurred and my time on the pitch had gone. Nottinghamshire chief exec Lisa Pursehouse was always hugely supportive and immediately told Luke that the club would pay me until the end of the season. That was a great gesture from Nottinghamshire at a time I really needed it. Luke always said how supportive Lisa was to my situation.

Great times. Great club. Nottinghamshire will always be a part of who I am.

Chapter 5

Retired Hurt

'Just fix me, keep me alive.'

Arrhythmogenic right ventricular cardiomyopathy, unsurprisingly better known as ARVC, is a rare disease of the heart muscle that causes it to thicken and makes the heart bigger. It's accelerated by exercise. There's no cure. If I carried on playing cricket there was every chance I'd drop dead. Full stops don't come any bigger than that.

The ECB advised caution on my retirement; they thought I was possibly being rash. They weren't keen on putting out such a closed book statement. They felt that while there was still the slightest chance, no matter how small, that I might still be able to play, that it might not be ARVC, it was the wrong course of action. They just wanted to say I needed to take the first half of the season off. But I wanted – needed – to put some closure on the situation. I didn't want to play this game of ifs and maybes. People said I was being led by emotion. Emotion? I nearly died. I'd lost the very thing that defined me. So yes, there was plenty of emotion. I was a young man utterly devastated. What I needed was some positive emotion. I needed a future, not a past. I didn't care how it looked.

The official announcement of my retirement came at 11.00 am the morning after the devastation. Luke did all the negotiations about statements and wording with the relevant press offices. Much of it he did through blurred vision. Both he and Lisa Pursehouse at Nottinghamshire were crying. As an agent, Luke could have been forgiven for trying to delay the announcement himself. It's hardly commercially wise to say a client is retiring. Most agents would try to drag the situation out. But Luke isn't like just any agent. Our relationship has always gone beyond that. We've known each other a long time, been through thick and thin together. He's said himself that he sees me as a little brother, and as such he could see that I needed, for my own sake, to draw a line under the situation. He understood me well enough to know it was that element of finality that would allow me to move on.

All of me was saying, 'Right, let's get this out there. I've hidden it for long enough', but a little bit of me was also wondering, 'Well, this is going to be interesting. I wonder what the fallout is going to be. I've been here a week now. I wonder what's going to happen?'

It was just carnage.

Within minutes, my phone was going mad. The announcement was a shock to everyone, even my teammates at Nottinghamshire. They'd heard rumours about my condition but nothing concrete. They had a meeting and a few of them were really upset, Stuart Broad among them, which I took as a massive compliment – Stuart Broad getting emotional about me?

My phone crashed again and again. The attention was unbelievable, but as a sportsman that's exactly what you like, so it helped enormously. At an incredibly tough time it was a great distraction. The negativity and hurt that I had to retire was suddenly weighed off against the welter of love that was coming my way. Peter Moores rang me, offering his sympathy, which shows the class of the man, as did assistant England coach Paul Farbrace.

'Farbs,' I said, 'this all your fault for putting me through the wringer with the T20 World Cup Final.' Two days before my attack, I'd watched England lose to the West Indies in the last over of a real epic nail-biter. 'The stress it put me under was too much.'

Farbs laughed. His was one of the voices I really treasured hearing. So positive, so encouraging. England one day captain Eoin Morgan was another who was really upbeat when he called. So many people for whom cricket meant everything could put themselves in my shoes. They asked themselves what they would want to hear – and then they said those words to me.

Olympic gold medallist and world heavyweight boxing champion Anthony Joshua tweeted me, as did the man with whom I suddenly had so much in common, Fabrice Muamba.

'Just take every day as it comes,' he told me. 'Sometimes you're gonna feel down and miss the game. Other days, especially when others pass from the same thing, you're gonna thank your lucky stars that you're here. Friends and family will help you through it.' He couldn't have been more right.

There were messages coming from all over the world. Former Australia captain Michael Clarke tweeted me: 'Absolutely devastated for you.' People say social media is damaging and negative, but for me it was a saviour. How could Michael Clarke, and pretty much everyone in the Indian Test team too, have messaged me if it wasn't for social media? In fact, when it comes to cricket, it would be easier to name the people who didn't message me than the ones who did.

Being an insecure kid, I used to lie in bed thinking, 'How many friends do I have? If I died, who would come to my funeral?' I would wonder who would miss me. I was so lucky because while I was still alive I saw what love I would get. And it was ridiculous. I had 20 million tweets about me in the first two hours. On occasions, it did feel like I had actually died. I saw a Sky News clip announcing, 'James Taylor has retired' in the same tone of voice as if someone had passed away. I was thinking, 'I'm still here lads!'

The tweets went on for days. It was so much of what got me through, the massive ego boost that I needed just at that time. Here I was, the lowest I could ever possibly be. I had so many dents, and these messages would knock them right out again. People would attach pictures of me batting for England. You might think that would have been hard at such a raw emotional time, but I actually liked it. It showed me doing what I did best. It showed me as a person who had achieved something, and hopefully entertained a few people along the way. I saved all of them.

Mick Newell said to me, 'I didn't realise you had any friends!' But I'm so glad I had that support. Every tweet was lifeblood for me, as important as the machine in my room when it came to keeping me going. Taking Jose and my family out of it, if there was one thing that changed everything it was social media. It saved my bacon. I was on my phone for hours and hours.

The deluge of goodwill didn't end there – it was the same at home. I had so many letters arriving it took me months to open them all. Luke's little twins Albie and Amelie sent me a toy lion – they said it was because I was as brave as one. I had it sleep with me while I was in hospital and I've still got it at home.

Strange what a small world we live in. Barely had the news broken than my dad received an email from a cricket correspondent in India. 'Get James over here. We've got the best people for hearts.' And he was genuine. That outpouring of love and support was as unbelievable as it was unexpected and it got me through the hardest time, the first three days after I realised my sporting life was over. It was such a warm feeling to know that I'd made an impression on people.

A lot of the time, people would sympathise with me, and the fact I was stuck in hospital, but I knew there was no alternative, and that knowledge made it a lot easier. At the same time, I couldn't help but have an eye on the cricket. In the second week, Nottinghamshire were playing Lancashire and I would have liked to have played against Jimmy Anderson after a long winter with him taking the piss. Instead I started to make a video diary to pass the time. 'I'm going to miss that duel,' I told the camera.

When it came to seeing old faces, I didn't need to step outside the hospital – the number of people who came to see me was incredible. One thing I hadn't quite reckoned on was how honest people were. Everyone who came through the door seemed to say the same thing: 'Shit, you look bad.' Up until that point I'd been consoling myself that I still looked all right.

England all-rounder Chris Woakes and his wife Amie are massive friends and had just got engaged when the initial incident happened. Normally we'd have been straight on the phone to them but we didn't want to burst their bubble. When Chris heard the retirement announcement, he wanted to leave the game Warwickshire were playing at Hampshire and drive straight up to the hospital. That wasn't an option, but as soon as he got back to the Midlands he came to see us, managing to sneak in a Nando's. Everyone who visited came in and sat by the end of the bed because that's where the chairs had been placed. Chris was different. He came straight in and pulled the seat right up to me. He was intensely concerned, like a brother would be. It was written all over his face. Then he started crying, which started Jose off crying – and then we all started crying. We were trying to eat this Nando's pretending we weren't crying. People must have been wandering past thinking, 'What the hell?'

They were so thoughtful. Amie's a beautician and the next time she came she wheeled her trolley in with all her files and products and did Jose's nails. It wasn't just Jose who got the treat. Chris brought me some shorts. We were so lucky we had our own room, but it was hot and I'd been in those same tracksuit bottoms for days. Shorts felt amazing.

Barely had we declared the news of my retirement than John Walsh, the main consultant for the cardio ward, who'd been on holiday, came in and introduced himself. He had a background in sporting cardiology and was keen to continue with my care.

'I've had a look at your scans,' he said, 'and there's a small chance that it's not ARVC.'

'What?'

Because of the unusual pattern of my presentation, John felt there remained a possibility of myocarditis, the cardiac inflammation caused by a viral infection. While my first MRI had shown my heart power was down and very much raised the suspicion of ARVC, a second MRI had revealed my heart was showing signs of improvement. If it was this underlying condition I'd had so long, why was it changing and improving? The results were put through another layer of expert analysis in London and they agreed there was a chance it could be myocarditis.

We leapt on this sudden glimpse of hope, convincing ourselves how this new possibility fitted the narrative of what had happened to me. It had to be a virus. This had never occurred before. What else could it be? How could I have operated as an elite level sportsman at the same time as harbouring a serious heart condition? How could a condition such as ARVC sit there benignly and then flare up out of nowhere? And why now? None of it made sense.

The fact it had happened in such an unimportant game was, for us at least, another pointer to it not being ARVC. How could it be? It was a totally non-stressful situation. We didn't realise that was the nature of the condition. It would have made no difference where I was when it happened. It wouldn't have mattered if I was haring between the wickets at Sydney running 3 to win a one day international. The point is, you're there, not how you got there. With ARVC, there are specific times, known as hot phases, when the disease is more dynamic, expanding the danger of sudden cardiac death. That chilly April morning in Cambridge, I was clearly going through a very hot phase indeed.

The more I learned about ARVC, the more I determined that I couldn't, mustn't, allow it in my life. ARVC, as Tim had stated, is genetic, passed down through the generations. If I carried the gene, there could be serious implications for those around me. When we came to start a family, it could affect mine and Jose's children. Also, if I did have the gene, who had I inherited it from? Did that mean other people in my family were potentially in danger? A genetics test would shed more light on the situation, but it would take months for a definitive result to come back. A whole sequence of genes would need to be analysed. It's that age-old question – how long does it take to look for a needle in a haystack? Clearly, I wasn't the first to be taken down this long and winding road. I was introduced to an inherited cardiac condition nurse specialist who talked me through the process and the potential repercussions before taking some blood and sending it off. It was one of those moments that reinforced how little control I had over my destiny. I'd gone from a person whose planning and preparation had been meticulous to someone who was a passenger in his own journey.

The odds of me being ARVC-free weren't in our favour. We hadn't known at the time, but right from the start, the considered opinion was the type of rhythm I'd experienced was suggestive of an underlying significant heart problem. Certainly, Tim was minded to think that way. He'd seen the initial heart readings taken when I came into A&E, and then again when my heart had returned to its normal rhythm. There were clear abnormalities on my resting heart trace that, in his mind, indicated that almost certainly I had an underlying condition. There was a high chance that a problem that had been storing up for years had now decided to show itself. When Tim carried out another ECG to measure the electrical activity of my heart and show whether or not it was working normally, the results only added to his suspicions. The pattern matched what would be expected from someone with ARVC. He didn't say anything at that point, but his view straight away was that my condition was probably going to end my career. An echocardiogram, which looks at the heart and nearby blood vessels, revealed subtle discrepancies that did little to dispel suspicions.

When it came to the full definitive picture, however, it was so hard for them to find out. I was a first. No one had presented at hospital in the state I was in, the main reason being that very few people could tolerate the rate and rhythm I experienced for any length of time. Long before they reached hospital they'd have lost consciousness. I was glad my fitness had saved me, but it was an unwanted first to add to my tally.

John kept my feet on the ground by telling me there was still a 90–95 per cent chance that it was ARVC. I appreciated that, but at this point I had one hell of a comeback in me. I'd retired, was never playing cricket again, never exercising again, was on the floor, thinking my life was over, and then someone had arrived on the scene and told me: 'Actually, it might not be what we think it is.'

When he said those words, everything changed. It was like there was light again. It had gone from 'Whoosh! Your life's over' to 'Hang on, there might be a chance'. Of course it was only an illness. My heart wasn't bigger because of ARVC, it was bigger because I was an elite sportsman who had trained and trained and trained.

All along I'd been harbouring glimmers that they'd got the original diagnosis wrong, that none of this could be correct, that somehow everything could somehow be made right again. Now it seemed that distant dream might be a reality. 'I knew those other doctors were wrong. I was right all the time.'

From nowhere I'd been offered a second chance. From it being 100 per cent my life as I knew it had gone, the odds had now turned, in my mind at least, to 40 per cent I'd be strapping the pads back on. Not that it was all shards of gold-tinted hope descending from the clouds. Another potential cause was also added to the mix – giant cell myocarditis, a rapid deterioration of the heart, which sounded brutal, awful, and uncontrollable. The medical profession know very little about it. Suddenly, ARVC didn't sound so bad!

As John spoke to us, all these new thoughts were rattling around in my head. Then he was paged – he was needed at a serious heart trauma. 'I've just to get this,' he said. 'I'll pop back in a minute.' He was the calmest man I've ever met. It was like he'd had a lunch interrupted. While he was away, a younger doctor who'd accompanied him said: 'I don't think it's ARVC.' It was the worst thing he could have done. John hadn't used those words. But this other doctor hadn't been anywhere near as measured. Throwing basic opinion into the mix, while good intentioned, can raise hopes unrealistically and set a patient up for another almighty crash. I'd raised my own high enough just on the back of what John had told me. I didn't need those expectations cranking up even higher.

Being in hospital made me appreciate doctors who can get news across with sensitivity. Yes, while further tests were being carried out it was a definite morale boost to think there might, just might, be a way back from the rockfall of bad news, but the basic standpoint was it was still by far most likely to be ARVC. The condition is, after all, exacerbated by exercise. I was always known for a very high level of gym activity and training, and then I stepped it up even more when I got into the international arena. Chances were that high level of activity exposed my genetic predisposition. On that basis, we were always up against the ropes. The only thing that allowed us to bounce back again and again was our positivity. Too many blows and we'd have been out for the count on the canvas.

John always spoke to us properly, like adults, and shared our positivity. Whatever it is you're telling a patient, just give them a little bit of love. There are ways of getting things across. John gave me a bit of optimism, not only in the sense of an alternative diagnosis but in terms of whatever was wrong with me being career changing rather than career ending. I could still coach, I could still go into business, I could still commentate, I could still take up another sport. However this turned out, it wasn't, John assured me, all doom and gloom. A lot of people die from ARVC – but a lot of people survive. He told me that the condition might progress rapidly and be difficult to control, but he would make me safe. He would ensure I was protected at all times. He wanted to get me back to living a full and active life. John gave me perspective, and that was something I carried with me throughout those days in hospital, and still carry with me now.

I'd be lying if I said positivity was my constant companion. All the time in hospital, I felt I had to keep any negative emotions in check, but it wasn't easy. Often I'd wake panicked in the night. 'I can feel my heart going!' It was a horrible feeling, having so little control over my body, a fear of what it might do, the dark and frightening place it might take me. Jose, as ever, was there for me. She'd sit on the bed and help me get back to sleep.

I always dreaded the next results coming – fingers crossed they'd be a little bit better than the previous ones. This continual mix of positive and negative, the lack of certainty, the rules of the game constantly changing, was really hard to deal with. I'd get to grips with one thing and then something else would happen and I'd have to get to grips with that. Some people talk about periods of their life as being like a rollercoaster. I'm not sure the rollercoaster has been invented that matched mine at that particular time. Every time I reached a sunlit peak of optimism, a rainstorm would appear to chase me down the other side. I'd hear the curtains being pulled back, the doctor would walk in, and I'd think, 'Oh my God. What are they going to tell us now?' I became so defensive of where I was on that rollercoaster, because one bad word and I'd be right back down at the bottom.

A basic anxiety about mortality was never far away, whether it be me feeling it or someone else. At one point my mum received an email from a doctor saying he needed to have a chat with us all – Mum and Dad, Jose and me. Essentially, everyone really close. It sent Jose into a panic. In her mind, there was only one explanation. 'Can no one else see what's going on here?' she was thinking. 'They're going to say that he's only got however long to live.'

She walked out and began searching for the doctor across the hospital.

'I don't want you telling James anything else,' she told him. 'He's had enough. We can't have any more bad news.' She genuinely thought we were going to be sat down and told I only had X many years left.

Thankfully, that wasn't the case. Although what he did want to talk to us about wasn't exactly the best news we'd ever had. When he mentioned blood clots, I felt sick to the stomach. Blood clots kill people, don't they? It's what happens to people on planes. It's what happens to very ill people on the verge of something terrible. But this was yet another offshoot of the attack I'd suffered. The trauma had caused blood to clot in the heart. That is a seriously frightening thought, yet another that made me feel a shiver down the spine – the cold steel of the sharp knife-edge of existence against my skin.

Tim's reasoning for gathering everyone together was to discuss the issue with the family all at once rather than explaining it again and again. It says everything for the mental strain we were under, the constant fear that the worst news was yet to come. All Jose could think when Tim began talking about blood clots – and thankfully he reassured us that the clotting wasn't life-threatening – was, 'Thank God!'

On another occasion, a doctor told us, 'We don't know when this is going to get worse. It could be six months, it could be six years, it could be sixteen years.'

We couldn't comprehend what we were hearing. For Jose, especially, it was just too much. 'I'm going to get some dinner,' she said quietly. She sat down against a pillar in the corridor and just screamed tears.

I needed to speak to John Walsh. 'James,' he reassured me, 'I've done all the stats with your heart and your life expectancy, while your heart rate remains as it is, should be that of an average man. This is not a death sentence. Chances are something else will get you first.' An odd thing to be punching the air about, but there you go. That's how quickly my life had switched round.

It was just one thing after another. We'd be at the top of the hill looking at the clouds disappearing, the sunlight coming through, and then next minute we'd be tumbling to the depths of the deepest dimmest valley – and we'd have been smashed again and again on the way down. Jose was forever aware of what this constant worry was doing to me and, as with the email to my mum, would challenge the situation – 'Right, enough's enough' – and sort it out. We were never going to be a passive part of the process. If something needed questioning or challenging, then that's what happened. She knew how important it was for me – for us – to remain positive.

If I'd not had Jose with me in hospital, I know darker thoughts would have been with me. Massively so. There were times, especially at night, when the sadness would overwhelm me, to the extent that if she hadn't been there I'd have been out the window. To lie there at night and know she was down there next to me was incredible. At the darkest point of my life she was my absolute saviour. Out of those sixteen days we were in hospital, Jose barely left my side. Once, her mum took her back to our house because she wanted to cook me some food and bring it back. When she got home, all she could do was cry. She was inconsolable. She didn't want to be there. She just wanted to be back with me. Another time, her family took her out to Wagamama for lunch. She was sitting, squashed between her brother and sister, not really wanting to be there, when I texted her a picture. It was of my old teammate Woody pushing me around outside. I'd not been out until that point, the doctors hadn't been too keen, but as soon as Jose was out the door our first thought was, 'Shall we?' The sense of freedom, the fresh air, the ripping away of the walls, was amazing. And being with Woody meant it was such good fun. It was a huge moment for me, a reminder of what it was to be in the open air, joking, messing around, having a laugh. When Jose got that picture it was the first time since the whole business started that she'd really smiled. I wish I'd seen it, but I'm glad I was the cause of it.

And that was it for separation. The rest of the time we were together. The nurses were unbelievable about it. Amazing. There was just one time a nurse told us off for being in the same bed. Jose was just giving me a cuddle on top of the duvet. But that was one time in sixteen days. They were incredible, so, so understanding. The same with visiting hours – they just weren't an issue; it was like a revolving door. The hospital staff were so accommodating. We must have had a hundred visitors. Broady came to see me, and Woody came in every day. He wouldn't come for ten minutes; he'd sit with me for two hours. Anthony Dyer, who runs a sports clothing brand in Nottingham, was another lifesaver. Every time he came he brought us a McDonald's. At the same time, his wife Laura would bring Jose a load of magazines. I used to be that bloke who, when faced with visiting someone in hospital, didn't want to go. Now I'd be straight there because I've experienced first-hand what a boost it is.

People like that were a breath of fresh air because they didn't act any differently. When someone nearly dies, everyone around them, consciously or otherwise, plays out a little video in their head. It's a video without that person in it. That's what causes the upset. Everyone who visited had clicked play on that video. They knew it, and I knew it. I'd watched it a hundred times myself. What you don't need, though, is a running commentary. It doesn't need constant analysis and I was lucky enough that so many of those close to me realised that. I rarely saw people's upset because they would hide it from me. I think anyone in hospital will say it can be very hard if people are constantly being sad for you and over sympathetic. I was sad. The tears came again and again. But that's all it was. It was never 'Why me?' I never allowed that internal conversation, and externally people were sensitive enough not to mention it either.

It's the same with doctors. Not everyone was as great as John and Tim. The odd one would come round with medical students and it felt like they were showing off in front of them. Once, before Woody took me, I asked if it was OK if I went outside. The reply was, 'Do you not understand how serious this is? You're not going anywhere for a while.' It was as if he thought I was stupid.

Students, meanwhile, would be asked to discuss my condition with the doctor. They'd be analysing readings on the monitor as if I wasn't there. It felt insensitive. It made me feel like a guinea pig.

Another time, Jose was pushing me in my wheelchair to a little café in the hospital and a doctor passed us, one we hadn't seen for a while. By this time, unless it was Tim or John, I didn't want to speak to anyone. Speaking to more doctors just kept muddying the waters. Jose was the same. She put her head down and kept pushing. It was no good. The doctor said she'd been looking at my scans.

'I'm so glad,' she said. 'It looks a happier heart now. When you came in I'd never seen a heart so unhappy.' She was talking about heart transplants and all sorts. It was well-meaning, obviously, but in our heads, the word 'transplant' was a reminder again of how delicate things were, how fragile. We didn't need those thoughts. We needed to keep our heads in as positive a place as possible. We'd made a safe bubble for ourselves and then all of a sudden it had been popped. Being in hospital, and being such a positive person, it was hard for me to deal with people whose job it was to tell me negative things. It becomes very easy to dislike someone in those circumstances, which I recognise can be unfair.

Down the years, I'd always been more naturally optimistic in character than Jose, but in those hard days in hospital her resilience and positivity really came to the fore. She kept saying this one line to me again and again: 'When life gives you lemons …' At first I didn't really understand what it meant. I'm still not 100 per cent sure! But in my heart it meant, 'When life knocks you down, you've got to crack on.'

If I hadn't had Jose, it would have been a whole different story. In tough times you need a lot of love, and she gave me so, so much love. I don't think I ever truly thought about jumping through that window, but I did wonder whether without all the love I had around me if I might be in a different frame of mind. If you don't have love around you, what do you have?

Thankfully, Jose had her own support network. Her mum, her brother and her sister stayed in our house for a week while I was in hospital. Jose's brother Campbell is a lawyer in London and he took a week off work just like that. It was amazing. That kind of support made the world of difference to both of us.

The room, meanwhile, was beginning to have a slightly more domestic feel. Cards from well-wishers had begun arriving at the house and Jose's family had brought them in and put them on the window ledge. We had bags of food and snacks, and even a plant of some sort had appeared. I was thankful for the window. It wasn't exactly a room with a view – all I could see was a grey hospital landscape, steam pouring into the sky – but it gave me something to look outwards at during a time of a lot of conspicuous inward looking. I was very fortunate to have my own room with a loo and a shower. I'm not sure how people manage on a ward in that situation. Whoever you are, having some privacy, some space for yourself and your loved ones, is vital. It's a place where so much absolute tumult can happen. Similarly, there are intensely personal moments of reflection. How that can be played out in front of other people I do not know.

I was still attached to a box twenty-four seven. If I was ever to escape it and get out of hospital, the doctors needed either to have a definitive answer to my illness or ensure I was entirely safe in the meantime while tests were completed.

One option was fitting the internal defibrillator I'd been shown at the time of the diagnosis.

'I'm not having that. That is not going inside me.'

Different issues were spinning around my head. I'll openly admit I was quite vain about the way I looked – I'd worked relentlessly to ensure I had a good body – so then to be cut open and have something the size of a mobile phone stuck in my chest was almost beyond comprehension. I didn't want a big scar. It felt like a massive ego dent. But as well as that, the thought of having something physically sat in my chest was awful. And anyway, I'd not received total 100 per cent confirmation that my problem was ARVC. What happens if it isn't? Does it have to come out again?

Another possibility was a biopsy, which would confirm whether it was ARVC or not virtually straight away.

'OK, get me into theatre!'

However, I should have known by now there was no such thing as a smooth ride. They'd say, 'We could do this and it would be a big step forward', and then would come the 'but …'. In this case the 'but' was the fact that the biopsy would have to be taken from the thinnest wall of my heart. There was a risk the forceps could penetrate the heart and cause serious damage, as well as dislodge the blood clot or cause my chest to need draining. John, understandably, wasn't keen.

'Is there anything else you can do?'

'Well, your last option is to have a life vest on. An external defib.'

'Brilliant!' Then I had another thought: 'What does it look like?'

But that was soon outweighed by the overall thought of 'Get me out of here!' At first, I hadn't wanted to be anywhere else. I knew I needed to be in hospital, so that made it easier. However, as time dragged on I was increasingly desperate to breathe some fresh air, have even the slightest taste of normality. There'd be talk of me going home, but then something else would crop up and it would go on a couple more days. I'd been in that hospital bed for two weeks. I needed to get out of there.

The life vest people came the next day with this bit of kit worth thousands. It was essentially a 5kg man bag with straps that went across my chest holding the pads that, in an emergency, would shock me, against my upper back. All the time it monitored my heart rate. If it felt the need to shock me, it would siren. If I didn't manually stop it in thirty seconds, it would send several hundred volts coursing through my body. It looked uncomfortable but on the other hand sounded a hell of a lot better than having a bit of metal shoved in my chest if I didn't need it.

They taught me how to put it on and emphasised again that the only way they could let me out of hospital was if I constantly wore it. At the same time, they did shove a small USB device in my chest to keep a track on my heart activity. That hurt – man, did it hurt – but it wasn't a defibrillator and to me at that time that's what mattered.

To celebrate my last full day in hospital, Jose went home and made me a lasagne with salad; to have a bit of Mary Berry dressing was such a treat. I said goodbye to the nursing staff, who had been so amazing. They were great with me right from the start and just got better as time went on – truly phenomenal, so giving and sensitive. In your darkest time, just to have people being nice to you means so much.

I put the life vest on, signed a few papers, and that was it. Sixteen days after warming up at Cambridge, I was going home.

Chapter 6

Out

I went into Nottingham City Hospital a professional cricketer with an England career. I left with a small bag of belongings and a defibrillator. I had no purpose, no structure, nothing.

My mum helped us clear out the hospital room and, with my life vest on and defib box hanging by my side, I climbed into the passenger seat of Jose's car and we drove home. I don't know what it's like to take a newborn baby home from hospital, but in the case of this particular journey that's how it felt – and I was the new arrival. Jose was cautious in the extreme, not wanting to rush, feathering the brakes, taking each turn desperately slowly. Eventually, however, there we were, back in our street.

Pulling up outside the house felt like a big moment. Finally, I was back home. But this was most definitely a beginning, not an end. Who could possibly say what the future looked like?

We'd always had a little routine. If I'd had a bad day at cricket, Jose would meet me at the door and close it behind me. We'd always joke that if she closed the door we wouldn't think about whatever had happened anymore. Cricket was left on the doorstep. From that point we could relax and be ourselves. If ever that tradition seemed appropriate then now was the time. So when we walked up the drive we made sure that I went through the door first and Jose, as ever, shut it behind me. We stood in the porch, with well-wishers' letters on the doormat, and hugged each other so tightly. We didn't need to say anything. The past sixteen days spoke for themselves. We both knew that perhaps we couldn't shut the door on this problem. It was a little bit bigger on this occasion. But we also both knew we'd give it our best shot.

After all the madness of the past two weeks, we didn't do much. In fact, so wary were we of my condition we were creeping around like old age pensioners for days. But it was great to get out of hospital and just go home and sit on a sofa and watch TV. A neighbour brought round some brownies her children had baked for us, and later we got ready for Jose's family and my mum to come over. I had a shower while Jose cooked. Never have I better appreciated normality. Well, normality of sorts – I would be in a life vest until the doctors could deliver a definitive diagnosis. And because the waters were still stormy I could never take it off. It was with me twenty-four seven.

I got fed up of it pretty quickly. I used to go in the shower just to get it off me. Sometimes I'd put a T-shirt on and go back downstairs without it on, hoping Jose wouldn't see. She'd either work it out because the straps weren't obvious or go mad when she found it lying on the bed.

On another occasion I was heading into town with Woody when it suddenly occurred to me that I'd got the vest but not the battery. Woody and I thought about it, and possibly we might have carried on if it weren't for one small matter – we were meeting Jose and, justifiably, she'd have gone mad.

The life vest was a huge inconvenience but a potentially lifesaving one. If there was a possibility that I wouldn't need an internal defibrillator in the long run, it was something I was willing to tolerate. 'If I don't need that thing in my chest,' I'd say, 'I'm not having that thing in my chest.'

Now I was out of hospital, requests came flooding in for interviews. Jose and I had talked about clawing something back from the situation by raising awareness of heart disease, and with all the attention on me it seemed a good opportunity. I decided to stage a press day. I did BBC, then Sky, and then a round table with the journos. They all said the same thing: 'It must be so hard to take, because you'd worked so hard to be an England cricketer.' And of course they were right. All I'd ever wanted to do was play for England. It was all I'd ever worked for, and then it was taken away. If I'd blagged my way there it might have been different. But I hadn't. I'd battled so hard to get to where I was. When they spelled it out so bluntly, I could feel the tears welling up. The truth they had identified was an obvious one – but it was still so raw, it still hurt. I was trying to hold my emotions back but it was difficult. For Luke, it was too much – he was crying at the back of the room. He stopped the interview and pulled me aside. 'Maybe we should stop. I'm not sure if this is helping.'

But I wanted to carry on. I went back in and finished it off. It had to be said, and it had to be faced; there was no point hiding away or postponing it.

Early on, I met ECB chairman Andrew Strauss and chief executive Tom Harrison in a coffee shop in Nottingham. They wanted to catch up and see how I was. Strauss was a man I had a lot of respect for, having made my England debut with him as captain. Harrison had always been very good with me too. They offered their genuine commiserations. I appreciated them making an effort to come and see me and we left it at that. Alastair Cook took time out of his busy schedule to visit me too, something that meant an incredible amount to me. He was so supportive, so positive. There was no way he was going to allow me to feel forgotten. He wanted me to know I was very much in everybody's mind.

'Is there anything we can do for you?' he asked. He'd obviously thought long and hard about that question, coming up with the idea of the England lads giving a percentage of their match fees to the British Heart Foundation. In no time at all, they'd donated £25,000.

For the first few weeks, Jose went everywhere with me. When I started doing interviews or filming, any small bits of work, she would come with me. She was my minder, nurse, girlfriend and carer all rolled into one. She took a term off school to do that. She gave everything to me, was my absolute and unshakeable support, and I'll never forget that. Early on we were invited on *Good Morning Britain*, the ITV breakfast show hosted by Piers Morgan and Susanna Reid. Jose wouldn't normally do anything like that, but the fact she'd been by my side for everything so far meant she agreed, albeit a little nervously.

Before they interviewed me, they showed some clips of me playing. Instead of the upbeat music that might usually play over the top of a highlights package, this was accompanied by something much more downbeat. As I watched, I could feel myself going. 'Oh God,' I was thinking, 'don't cry.' At the same time, the narration was saying really lovely things about me. I was welling up. Added to that, Piers makes guests feel like he wants a bit of reaction. His first question wasn't exactly subtle. It was, essentially, 'You've lost everything. You must be gutted.' On the other hand, that was pretty much a fair summary of the situation.

It wasn't just me, though – we were all coming to terms with what had happened. It hit my dad quite hard, because he knew how difficult the next stage would be, living a life away from what I loved. There's a strange symmetry between me and my dad. He too had just had his best ever season when he was forced to finish. A fall at Southwell saw him dislocate and break his hip and back. He came round in the ambulance room and eventually paramedics came and took him away. They dropped my dad at the hospital in Newark, where he was expecting surgery, only to be told they didn't have an anaesthetist. He then had to wait for another ambulance to take him from Newark to Nottingham. By the time he arrived it was 9.00 pm, all with his hip out of place. It was six hours before they operated on him. Every minute that passed was just making things worse. He was then transferred to a hospital in Sheffield for another two months. He describes it as being written off as though he was dead. Three decades on and there he is in another hospital watching the same thing happening to his son.

I was determined not to sit around and mope and so we'd go out with me wearing the life vest. What I hadn't reckoned with was its unnerving habit of talking if it felt something was wrong. If it felt my heart do something unusual, it would speak up in a satnav woman's voice: 'Preparing to shock!' It did make us laugh.

It did it in a couple of restaurants, also at Trent Bridge when I went down to watch the cricket, and Nottingham Forest, the latter being the first outing I'd had without Jose.

It would throw in a siren as well, not quite as loud as a fire alarm but not far off, to warn the shock was on its way. I knew the pain would be like nothing I'd ever felt before and was thankful I was able to manually override the machine. Trouble is, afterwards I'd be thinking, 'Why has it done that? It's done that for a reason.' The automatic instinct, knowing a horrible shock was coming, was to override. Then, on reflection, I'd be thinking, 'Well hang on, maybe it was trying to tell me something.' Most of the time, though, I just considered it to be either wrong or oversensitive; a piece of temperamental rubbish going off all the time.

I was never embarrassed when the alarm went off, but it was a big switch from my early thoughts of not wanting anyone to see me that way. On *Good Morning Britain*, they asked me to show the defib on camera. They wanted me to unbutton my shirt. Vain old me might not have been too keen but now I saw it as part of a necessary transition. I knew it was going to be hard enough dealing with my new circumstances as it was without battling with myself as well – I might as well just front up and say exactly how it is.

One thing I hadn't reckoned on was security. The terrorism alert was at its highest, and nothing looks more like a suicide belt than a portable defibrillator. Not only have I got a box full of wires hanging off my shoulder but I've got straps all across my upper half and two big metal pads on my back. Jose used to dread us getting stopped on the Tube, but because I wasn't used to having the device with me it was automatic for me to walk on without even thinking. More than once I'd stand up to get off and it would drop on the floor. We'd laugh about it. What else could you do? We always tried to make a joke of any weird occurrence if we could.

At high profile sporting events it was inevitable I'd be searched, but that hadn't actually occurred to me until we went to a rugby match at Twickenham. There were two security guards on the turnstile. As the first started patting me down, the other chap looked across. Immediately, he recognised me and looked at his colleague – 'Just don't.' He took away his hands and I was good to go. That happened a couple of times at Twickenham but because there's a bit of crossover between cricket and rugby fans, and also I'd been all over the press at that point, people knew who I was and it never became an issue.

Twickenham is a magnificent stadium, but not if you've got a recently diagnosed debilitating heart condition. When we went to the England v Wales game, we had tickets near the top of the stand. Every set of stairs went straight up. Stair after stair after stair. It was tough. I got to the top and I could feel my heart racing. 'Oh shit,' I thought, 'it's going to happen again.'

I turned to Jose. 'I'm going to have another heart attack. I can feel it coming on.'

There's no scarier feeling than when your heart goes haywire. It's being on the edge of life with no control over whether you're going to plunge over the side. Thankfully, Jose helped me calm myself, but on the way home in the car I was mulling it over in my head. I, a man who'd always prided himself on being the fittest of the lot, had walked to the top of a stand at Twickenham and it had nearly killed me. That kind of thing brings you right back down and knocks your confidence. I just broke down.

'I'm not invincible anymore,' I wept. It had taken me almost two months to reach a simple realisation – I wasn't that person anymore. That man who could do anything he put his mind to. That man who could defy the odds and make anything happen. That man who could overcome hurdle after hurdle. I was a different person – delicate, fragile. I'd gone from granite to glass. When you're used to being invincible, that's tough. It recalibrates everything you've ever thought about yourself.

Jose pulled into a service station. She wanted us to get out of the car. 'Come on, Jim, let me hug you properly.' She wanted to hold me tight, shield me from the world.

'No, not here. I can't have anyone see me like this.'

I couldn't face the thought of anyone witnessing the new non-invincible me – defenceless, weak, vulnerable. The tears kept coming. Mine and hers. I just couldn't believe it.

Persuading those around me that I would be all right on my own was another challenge. Understandably so – when you've cheated death, people are bound to build a protective barrier around you. The instinct is not to let anything into that bubble that might provide a threat. It's amazing to be on the end of that kind of love, but for me there was a growing element of wanting to get some independence back and do things on my own.

Early on, Luke tried to instil some order back in my life. Practically overnight I'd gone from 'Eat now!' 'Wear this!' 'Play now!' – preseason, end of season, winter tour – to nothing. He set up a Google calendar that we could both access. On it, we'd put everything, be it a hospital appointment or my mum coming round. He reckons without that calendar I'd still be wandering round in my underpants.

Some days, I'd walk down to Trent Bridge. It wasn't easy. At this stage, such was the muscle wastage, going from an extreme sporting lifestyle to being in a hospital bed for sixteen days, and then doing nothing at home, that my legs were hurting after a 200-yard walk. At the same time, the support from people walking down the street was unbelievable. In fact, the attention never really died down. It was relentless for six months. Wherever I was, I got so much more attention than I ever did before, partly because of what I did in South Africa, but I think mainly because of the illness.

I could see the quandary playing out in people's minds. Should everyone be glad I am alive? Or should everyone be sad I can't play cricket? I was aware that people didn't know how to react to what had happened. And in all honesty, at that point I wasn't too sure myself. While people naturally assumed my diagnosis was all cut and dried, I was still waiting for the definitive result. Yes, I had retired, and yes I had ARVC, but that was only a 98 per cent diagnosis. I was always clinging on to the 2 per cent. The fact that I was still harbouring hopes, nobody knew.

People would stop and console me, offer their commiserations, or just give me a smile and a 'hello'. They understood exactly what I'd lost. They knew what it meant to me. And they knew how close I had come to not being here at all. For someone whose life had vanished, and was worrying if they might perhaps vanish with it, those little hellos were like mountains of reassurance. The letters and social media messages were the same. At a time when all I could think was how horrendous I looked, losing my muscle and putting on weight, they really kept me going. Everyone pumping me up was compensation for me, feeling like and, in my eyes, looking like shit.

Going back to Trent Bridge was a little bit embarrassing. I was used to being the picture of health, one of the fittest, if not the fittest, in the dressing room. Now the body I'd worked so hard for was propped up by a life vest. There was no escaping the facts of what had happened. I was, after all, carrying a big bloody house brick full of wires around with me. I sat in the dressing room. I loved it, being back around the boys, watching them out in the middle. But even then, because my heart was so bad at that point, and so, so sensitive, watching wasn't always good for me. I was the only person in the ground who didn't want the game to be exciting.

There was possibly one other person in sport who knew that feeling, and I still had the life vest on when I was asked to speak to Fabrice Muamba as part of a BBC documentary. The first time we met on the programme was the first time we met full stop. It was a big moment. Those who suffer from any serious condition will tell you how heartening – no pun intended – it is to meet others who know exactly what it is to suffer because they have been through the same experience. Fabrice had the same condition, except his went the next step. He was basically dead and only the work of the medics at White Hart Lane, allied to the hospital facilities nearby, saved him. Perhaps neither of us should be on this Earth right now, but that applies in particular to Fabrice.

With a broad smile, he took hold of my hand and shook it. He was a lovely bloke – infectiously upbeat while at the same time being fairly reserved. He would never joke about ARVC, whereas my default position is always to make light of things, to put other people at ease as much as me. I would often say to people, 'Oh, I'd better not do that or I'll have another bloody heart attack!' That was not Fabrice at all. But our different characters didn't matter; what mattered to me was meeting the living embodiment of light at the end of the tunnel, and to see someone who'd lost so much carry himself so well. As someone, like me, to whom fitness had meant so much, he also talked to me about staying healthy going forward. Weights, for instance, disagreed with him. As someone so conscious about staying fit, I found that insight fascinating.

For seven weeks, we had the hope it wasn't ARVC. I clung on to it like a passenger on a sunken ship clinging to a piece of wreckage. I didn't dare let go. I didn't want to drown.

Still I couldn't understand why, if I had this potentially longstanding heart condition, it hadn't happened until that day. I also couldn't comprehend why now I felt my heart's every little flicker, every little misbeat, when I'd never noticed before. Surely if I had something as big as ARVC I'd have felt it. People say I'm now hyperaware of my heart's activity because I've suffered a major incident. I get that, but I still think I would have noticed.

When, finally, the tests were all done, it was John Walsh who called us into hospital to deliver the news. We'd had meetings with him before but this was the big one. We'd always be nervous on these occasions. Sat in an empty corridor waiting, Jose used to pop the tension by making me read out information leaflets to her. She found it hilarious because I hated reading out loud and would stumble over words. One time we hadn't realised John had appeared and was just stood there watching. We must have looked mad but it became our little routine.

This time, John waited in the room where the meeting was to take place. 'It's not good,' I turned to Jose as we walked in, 'he has a defib in his hand.'

John gave us the news. I was right. It wasn't good. It was, as they'd always thought, ARVC. And yet even then it wasn't absolutely, without doubt, 100 per cent clear. There was still a 0.03 per cent chance of it not being the condition. I was still clinging on, even if it was by the very end of my fingernails.

The night before the defib went in, John rang to say a colleague had seen the scan and the chance of it not being ARVC had gone up. Also, at this stage, we were still awaiting the result of a test to ascertain whether I had the ARVC gene. So there we were, the night before the operation, still discussing whether we wanted it to go in or not. John, though, was adamant. 'You need this in, no matter what. If it comes out again in five years, fine, but you need it in at the moment.'

It was all the confirmation I needed. 'Right, OK, I've got my head round it – it's going in.' Jose wasn't quite so sure. She didn't know if I should do it. But I'd made my mind up. I wanted it in.

Even so, it was tough to get my head around having something physically fitted inside my body. I didn't enjoy the thought of being cut open. When people talk about open-heart surgery, it is pretty terrifying. If I hadn't made that firm decision that it was the right thing to do, it would have been easy to waver. But I was positive and worked the rationale out. If something needed to be done, let's just get on and do it. The defib offered the reassurance of protection. If there was an issue with my heart, the pacemaker would try to bring the heart rate down and then if that didn't work it would give an electric shock, the idea being it would deliver it before I blacked out or was incapacitated.

The surgery lasted three hours. It would have been quicker but because I love the gym and had worked so hard, it took Tim Robinson forty minutes longer than usual to get through my pecs. In fact, the thickness of my muscle meant I needed a general anaesthetic. I didn't need to have the defib hidden beneath my muscle but I made the decision that, although it added complication to the procedure, it was preferable to it being visible just under the skin. The added layer of complexity bothered Jose and she pleaded with me to consider the simpler option, but I was adamant.

'I'm in my twenties, Jose. I want to be able to take my top off.' It's vanity, I know that. But I had lost so much; I didn't want to lose anything else. The way I'd changed physically was already a big ego dent. At first when I was in hospital I'd always have my top off because of all the wires. But after a week of not going to the gym I couldn't wait to get my top back on again. In my mind, I looked horrendous.

I was always used to seeing myself in the mirror and thinking I looked good, but as time went on I saw that muscle fading away. Feeling good and looking good was how I was so confident. To have that taken away hurt.

I came out of theatre with two electrode wires screwed into the wall of my heart. The wires from the electrodes ran back through a vein and into the defib itself. It is actually possible to see the wires running along the top of my chest but the defib itself is hidden, as I wanted, beneath my muscle. Tim did a fantastic job. You have to look very hard to see any sort of asymmetry.

It's major heart surgery to have a defib fitted and yet initially when I came round from the anaesthetic I felt fine. I was a little groggy, but that was it. Soon, though, it turned into the worst hangover ever – a terrible headache, and I was sweating so much. I was wheeled across to X-ray on the other side of the hospital to check the screws were in the right place, Jose trying to keep up alongside an enthusiastic porter who was doing a fair lick along the corridors. All was as it should be, but my misery and pain continued. The doctors offered me morphine but my mum pointed out that whenever she'd had it she'd felt sick. No way did I want to feel sicker than I already did, so I refused. Eventually, the feeling subsided, and I left the hospital – in Jose's blouse because I had my arm in a sling and I needed a button top. I was in great spirits, so happy not to have had to stay overnight and showing off the sizeable cut and stitches to Jose's mum, and enjoying her reaction. It was the biggest mistake I ever made – not wearing Jose's clothes; I'm talking about coming home. Initially, I felt fine, even more so when Jose and her mum made my favourite meal of pasta with a special home-made sauce. Then as soon as I climbed into bed, things took a massive turn for the worse. I began to feel absolutely terrible all over again – sweating, nausea, absolute sheer discomfort. The painkillers had started to wear off and I was so sore. My heart was obviously reacting to the operation too, racing away with itself. If it had been doing somersaults during the original event, now it felt like it was doing backflips, forward rolls, the lot. I was absolutely terrified. Jose and I rang the hospital twice telling them what was going on. They reassured us it was entirely normal given how close it was to the op. It was a horrible night, and one that felt so unfair. The defib was supposed to be a step forward, a big leap towards something resembling normality, and yet here we were in the dead of night once again clinging on to each other in fear. It felt all too familiar. All too much like it had before. Would this condition ever let us go? Ever allow our minds to clear? Ever allow us to gaze across clear water?

After three days I saw the England doctor and he gave me some proper hardcore painkillers. But that entire area was so sore. Also, for the next six weeks I had to remember something very important – if I lifted my left arm above shoulder height it would yank the defib wires straight out of my heart. When you think about how often you stretch without thinking, that's not as easy as it sounds. A further complication was another blood clot. Blood thinner was prescribed, adding another layer to my mental turmoil. What happened if I had an accident? Even a minor car crash would leave me screwed because I could just bleed out. It was for the same reason that I couldn't get into coaching earlier. If I'd been hit by a cricket ball on my heart after the operation, it could have caused serious damage. Add in the bleeding that comes with blood thinners and it could have been catastrophic.

For several days, I just retired to the sofa. It was a very flat period. Physically and mentally I was battered and bruised. Sometimes there's only so much a person can take and if there was a point I did start to recede into myself a little then that was it. Jose was the same. Her mum would come in and make us something to eat and we'd barely acknowledge it. It was a short time when the sun went in and the clouds came out.

The clouds, though, were gradually disappearing alongside the pain and discomfort, and, as our mood began to rise, I felt I was coming back to life. It was just five days after the op when, as we'd promised ourselves, we had a day out at Ascot, where I'd been invited to award the prizes after one of the races. I invited my old school pal Griff, and Amie Woakes came along with Jose. I went to present the prize, leaving the others in the parade ring with a lot of the press. I was a little wary of them being bothered and before I went mentioned that if any journalists came asking questions not to give them too much. No sooner had I headed off than a reporter was straight over, asking Jose how she had cared for me, how I was coping, and how our new life was shaping up. She was doing her best to brush him off and so he turned to Griff.

'Had a nice lunch?' the reporter enquired.

'Yes thanks, mate.'

'What did you have?'

'Beef.'

Griff was so proud of this little white lie – we had in fact had chicken – and his joy was confirmed a few days later when Amie found a *Daily Mail* article detailing mine and Jose's day out.

'On Wednesday,' read the piece, 'they had a slap-up meal in the Royal Enclosure — beef for mains. Taylor chomped it down.' It was so stupid but so funny. We laughed so hard and for so long. We hadn't laughed like that for ages. Everything was back in balance.

It was great to be back out in the real world, going to one of the great sporting occasions. With Ant and Dec, I was one of only three non-royals giving out prizes. As it turned out, the winner of my race was the great Frankie Dettori and he came up to the podium and gave me a big hug. I'd been speaking to Princess Anne as I waited to give Frankie the award, and then immediately afterwards was called over to do an interview with Clare Balding on Channel 4. On the way, I found myself having a two-minute chat with the Duke and Duchess of Cambridge. We talked about my other duty – picking the best turned out horse. Afterwards, we had a few hours with Ant and Dec and they were lovely blokes, exactly as you'd imagine them to be – best mates, really down to earth. In five days I'd gone from the operating theatre to the ultimate social whirl.

After all we'd been through, it meant a lot to Jose and me to have a day like that. I look at the photos and I can see how rough I was feeling. I was still incredibly tired and sore from the operation. In fact, if I'd properly comprehended how ill I really was, I don't think I'd have done it. It wasn't just the strain of the day, although it didn't feel a huge strain at the time, it was the fact of being in a crowd. The operation was so recent and the repair so tender that any knock in that area could have been a real setback. Even now, whenever I'm in big crowds, such as in a sports stadium or a bar, I will walk with my right hand over the left side of my chest as protection. If anybody knocks me above my defib it will really hurt.

Being out in such a busy place could be a double-edged sword. The attention, the positivity, and the sincere wishes of 'Good luck!' were incredible, such a boost, and 99 per cent of people were brilliant: 'How are you doing?' 'You were my favourite player', 'I loved that catch you took, that innings you played' – really positive. But that euphoria could vanish at any moment with something more negative. I could have been having the nicest day, my head in a good space, an escape from thinking about ARVC, and then all of a sudden someone would say something like 'You must be heartbroken', and I'd be right back down to earth.

Sometimes people would approach the matter by trying to relate to me – 'My granddad has got a defib'. And I'd think, 'Well, you just said it right there, mate – your granddad'. I was twenty-six.

The only time it ever got too much was at a one day international at the Oval that we'd been invited to. Literally hundreds of people were trying to relate their stories to us. Again, it was all really well meaning, and it sounds awful to complain about it, but on that particular occasion it became exhausting. In the end we just had to leave. I love talking about what's happened, but find it difficult when the conversation becomes draining. Even if it's not intended that way, it can feel like you're being bombarded by negativity and I neither want nor need that.

The cricket lovers I met were never insensitive – they weren't to know what was going on in my head. The same couldn't be said of Dominic Cork. At T20 Finals day I was doing a Q&A with Chris Woakes in front of 400 people when the ex-England all-rounder came up to me, when I had a microphone in my hand, mid-speaking, put his hand on my heart and said, 'Oh, still beating! I can vouch for that.' I didn't want to make a big deal of it in front of people, but inside I was thinking one thing: 'You twat'.

It was the first Q&A I'd done since I had my defib fitted. The unknown of the situation meant my heart was already performing somersaults. I had anxiety bouncing up and down through my body – shooting from my head to my toes and back again – the weirdest feeling. For him then to embarrass me like that put me right on the back foot. Bear in mind this was in front of 400 people. If anybody had been looking at me they would have been wondering what the hell was going on. Instead of standing still, I was agitated, moving around trying to find a drink to calm me down, somewhere to sit. I was beyond worried that my defib was going to go off, and all the time trying to answer questions. I was two seconds away from walking off. I was meant to do three more Q&As that day after that and I had to cancel them.

I'm more than happy to talk about my condition, but as soon as someone is disrespectful, that's different. This is an ongoing condition. Putting a defib in isn't a cure. That summer, in particular, I was experiencing endless physical and mental torment. One time I was sat in a restaurant with Mum and Dad and my heart started doing somersaults. I thought I was going to be sick, like I was going to have another heart attack. It was as bad as I've felt since the incident itself. I had to get out of there. I just got up, left, and went to sit in the car. My parents paid the bill and followed me out. Until then, my mum hadn't realised how badly it affected me day to day. That particular incident was exacerbated by my having a bad cold; illness always makes my heart more fragile. Since then she worries more. So to think the situation with my heart can be made a joke of is just crass. I can make a joke about if I want. That's my privilege. The same for others who know me well enough, just like friends will have a laugh and a joke if a pal breaks their leg. They do that because they know the person, they understand the boundaries. They know when to stop.

Remember also that I wasn't just thinking about myself. ARVC is a genetic condition. If I had it, then chances were that other people in my family had it too. That could be my dad, my mum, sister, cousins, anyone. That was what I was dealing with. It felt at times like there was a bullet ricocheting round a room waiting to strike any one of them.

Test Match Special asked me if I fancied doing a bit of commentary, and it was while I was working on a game at Northampton that I had a call from the hospital back in Nottingham. It was a genetic nurse. She might as well have hung up there and then; I knew exactly what she was going to say.

'You've got the ARVC gene,' she confirmed.

'OK, right – thanks.' Well, what else was there to say? I'd got the gene. Finally, I knew for sure it was ARVC. 'I can deal with that,' I thought.

But she hadn't finished. 'You've got another faulty gene.' I was sat in the commentary box and I just slumped. The whole process, right from the start, had been smashing me left, right and centre. Now this was like being on the floor with someone stamping on me. Someone large, heavy, and totally unforgiving.

She told me they'd found a rogue gene that had malfunctioned. It was the combination of the two genes that was causing the ARVC. The upshot was it would be harder for our siblings to be tested, or our children, because the geneticists wouldn't be looking for one gene, they'd be looking for a combination of two. I then had to go back on commentary and just get on with it.

Jose spoke to the same nurse. After all we'd been through together, all the turmoil, the ups and downs, the days in the hospital, the endless doctors coming in and out of the room, at the actual moment when we found out the inarguable truth that it was definitely ARVC, I was in a commentary box in Northampton and she was at home on her own. It seemed unnatural, strange. If ever there was a moment we should have been side by side it was then.

The final, somewhat drastic, confirmation I needed the defib came just weeks later. At this point, I had no clear knowledge of what my financial future looked like. While I was still recovering, I was doing bits and pieces of work as and when it was offered. I was conscious that it wasn't in my interests just to disappear. This particular Friday, I'd already done four hours' filming at Lord's to make a bit of cash when I got in a car to Leicestershire to do a half-hour Q&A followed up by commentary on the club's game that night – a bit of money here, some more there, and some more tagged on the end. It was a hectic day, and after the filming at Lord's I was stressing all the way back to Leicester. The minutes were ticking by because it was Friday evening and the traffic was bad. All the time I was thinking, 'I'm going to be late.'

Eventually I arrived at Grace Road, rushed across the car park, into the function room, climbed straight on stage, grabbed the mic, and started the Q&A with my former Leicestershire teammate Matthew Boyce. Inevitably, conversation quickly turned to my defib. There I was, laughing and joking, explaining what it was like to be at the mercy of a machine in my chest, when my vision started going blurry. I'd barely had time to register the change when 'Boof!'. Everything went black and I shot backwards across the room. I didn't know what had hit me. The first thing I remember was shouting, 'Fuck!' After a couple of seconds, I realised my defib had gone off. Because the scar was so fresh, the power should literally have exploded my chest open.

Two hundred people were staring at me. The sound of the deifb activating had amplified down the mic, like a stick of dynamite going off, to the extent that people had even heard it outside the room. Blown back several paces, somehow I'd remained on my feet. I tried my best to crack a joke.

'If you want to know what a defib going off looks like,' I told the audience, 'you've just seen it.' People laughed and there was a big round of applause. In all honesty, I couldn't believe that I could speak.

'That was amazing,' I added. At which point I picked up my bag and left.

I might have looked casual, but inside I was shitting myself. I went into the club offices to escape the crowds, chill, and sit down. I didn't know what this meant. In my head, I'd effectively had another heart attack. Thankfully, it being a match day, the Leicestershire doctor was on hand and he looked after me. The girls in the office sat with me too, checking all the time if I was OK. I felt so angry.

'It shouldn't have happened,' I kept repeating. 'It shouldn't have happened.'

At the same time I was taken aback by how the defib had actually activated, what it was capable of doing, the power, the force it had.

Boycey came to see that I was OK. He told me that all the time I was talking he could see the stress in my face. My pulse was clearly visible, flickering frantically beneath my eye. And then 'Bang!' off it went. The force, the power, was unbelievable. I couldn't believe it had happened. Trying to take a positive out of it, at least I knew my body – my new body – and what it was capable of a little bit better. It was a terrible thing to happen but it was a blessing because it said for sure that I needed a defib. In a very horrible way, it was the ultimate confirmation I needed.

I was meant to be commentating but obviously I cancelled. In the meantime, Jose and my mum drove across to see me. When they arrived, I was sat in a corner surrounded by people who probably didn't really know what to say. They hadn't expected this to happen any more than I had, and they were as lost as I was in the aftermath. Jose rushed straight across the room and held my head to her so tightly. I wasn't going to show it in front of other people, but I was lost and scared and wanted to cry, and she knew it. I felt helpless, clinging on to her for my life.

We left Grace Road and drove over to the hospital in Nottingham – in a car with Jose and my mum and a dodgy heart heading for a hospital in Nottingham. Where had I seen this before? We walked down those same familiar corridors and back on to the unit. Naïvely, I don't think any of us had anticipated being back there quite so soon – if ever.

John Walsh came in to reset the defib even though he was off duty in the gym at the time. 'I know how frightening it can be the first time,' he explained. John looked through the data. My heart, it transpired, had been racing at around 275 beats per minute. We were hoping he would say it was an inappropriate shock, that the defib shouldn't have gone off. Unfortunately not. It was purely down to stress. I was just stood still, talking, but the build-up, the combination of being stressed about being late, already having done four hours at Lord's, then rushing to the venue, had sent my heart rate through the roof. Readings later showed that when I got into the function room at Leicester, my heart was already at 130 beats per minute, and from that point on it never stopped rising, eventually peaking, within a minute, at 275, which it carried on doing until my defib kicked in.

I turned to Jose. 'This is really going to affect me, isn't it?'

It was a moment where we both suddenly understood that this was going to recur. We'd battled through so much, but that didn't mean ARVC intended to leave us alone. It wasn't something we could ever forget about. It would be with us forever.

My mood wasn't hugely improved when John told me the fact that the defib had gone off would mean I was barred from driving. After the travails of the past few months, I'd lined up a new Mercedes for a treat; now I was going to have to cancel. Jose had a different way of looking at it.

'Why don't you get the car, Jim?' she said, 'and just insure me on it instead?'

I knew exactly what she was angling for. It made me smile and we were back in our world again.

Knowing you have something inside your body capable of that kind of power, that kind of shock – abrupt, violent, painful, distressing – is deeply unnerving. It's not like having your arm in a sling, or your foot in plaster.

I'm not saying physical injuries aren't bothersome and unpleasant, but there will inevitably be times when you forget, perhaps caught up in conversation, or watching a film on TV. When it's your heart it's different. We define ourselves by our heart. Emotionally, physically, it is the very essence of who we are. The heart is at the epicentre of poetry and song for a reason. It is a symbol of strength and love, the source of life itself. Consciously or subconsciously, it is an absolute constant in our minds. Just think about any time you have suffered palpitations, or the sickening heart-wrenching experience of turbulence on a plane, or the adrenalin injection of a shock of a traffic accident or whatever. One way or another, the heart will let it be known it's there. For someone with ARVC, this is amplified a hundred times. If your heart is background noise, turned down to one, mine is in surround sound clarity on ten. That means when something does go amiss, the emotional reaction – the panic, the fear – is accentuated by the same amount again. It's a terrifying place to be, like sitting alone in a cinema watching your own worst nightmare on a massive high definition screen – a nightmare likely to reach out and pluck you from your seat and throw you into a maelstrom of torment at any moment.

I never quite knew when I was going to be handed a ticket to that particular cinema show, but an occasion soon cropped up when Jose and I went to stay at Amie and Chris Woakes' place. It's always a great evening when the four of us get together. Amie had cooked for us all and we had the usual fun before Jose and I headed up to bed. We were just drifting off when out of nowhere my heart began to turn somersaults, beating super fast in what felt like a horribly irregular rhythm. I sat up, slung my feet over the edge of the bed, and braced my arms against the mattress. I was breathing hard, sweating, desperately trying to deal with what was happening. Forget living by the minute; in those situations you live by the nanosecond.

Jose sat up; she knew exactly what was happening. This wasn't the first time. She scrambled over to me and I held her hand to my heart so, wordlessly, we could be in the same space. Neither of us knew where that space would take us next, but the most obvious place was somewhere including a huge electric shock.

'The defib will kick in?' I whispered to Jose.

'Yes,' she calmed me, 'the defib will kick in. It's just a shock. It's just a shock.'

She got me to lie down and curled up and hugged me from behind. I was bracing for the shock and she was too. My head was pushing into the pillow, and, no hiding it, my face was screwed up with fear. We were both so utterly

Clearly a fashion guru even
aged 1.

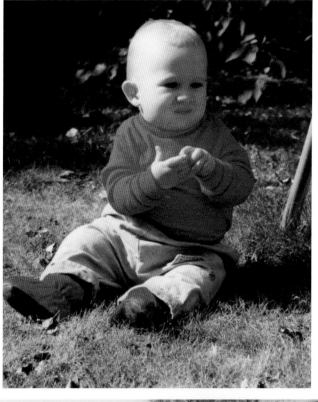

Family photo with Mum,
Dad and Sarah at a cross
country event.

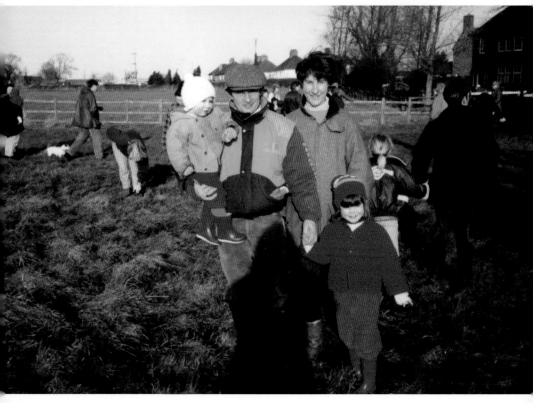

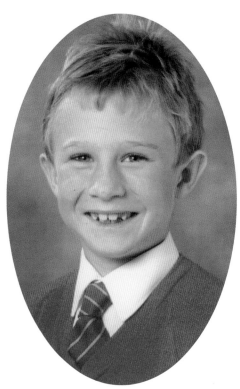

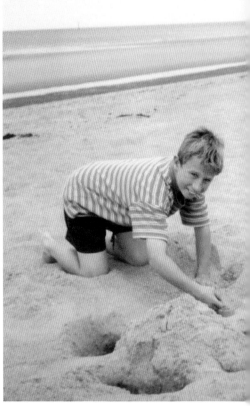

My first school photo aged 7 (pre-braces!).

Building sandcastles on my favourite beach in Lincolnshire, Sandilands Beach.

I made the fence look a lot taller than it was! Competing in a cross country event, aged 5.

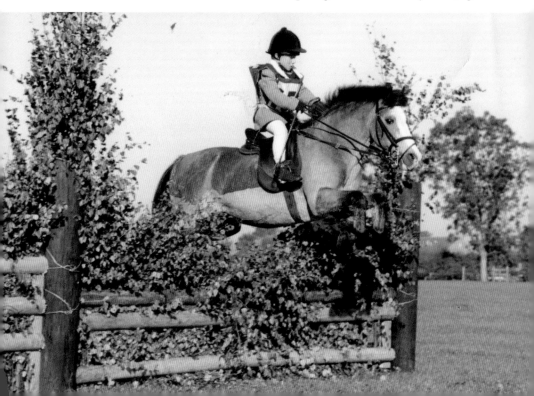

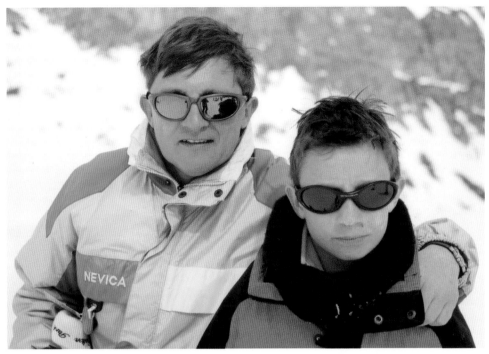

Dad and I trying to look cool with our shades while skiing in France (aged 8).

My first catch! Aged 11, catching a 4lb Rainbow Trout.

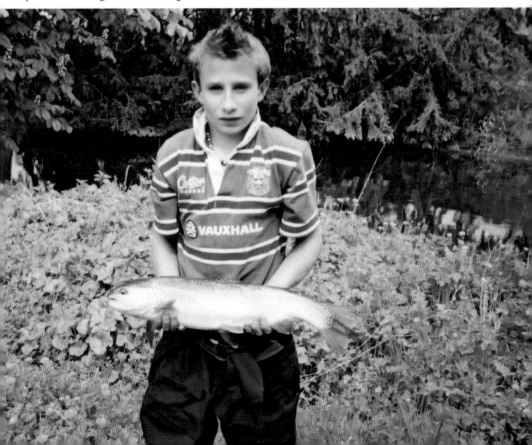

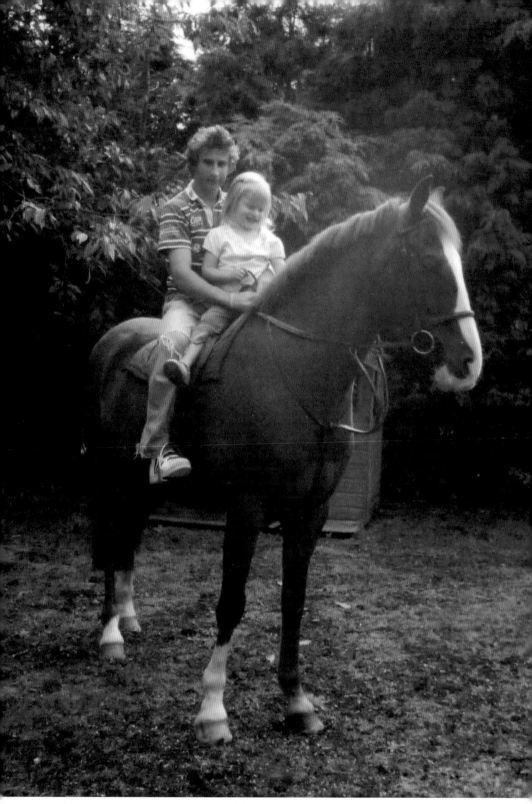

Madeline Schofield and I riding Mum's horse at home in Leicestershire, aged 14.

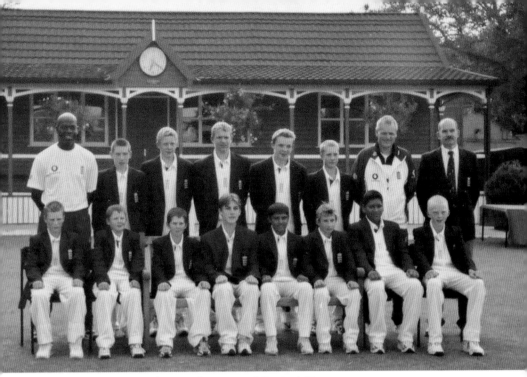

Midlands Under 13s team photo at the Regional Festival, Taunton.

Being presented my Midlands Under 13s cap by Andrew Caddick.

My first day with England Under 15s at the ECB National Academy and they didn't have any small sizes.

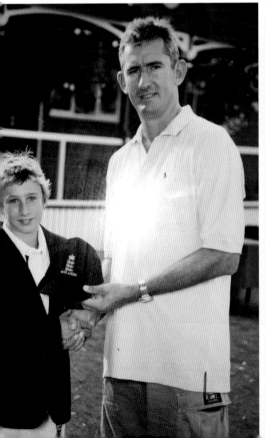

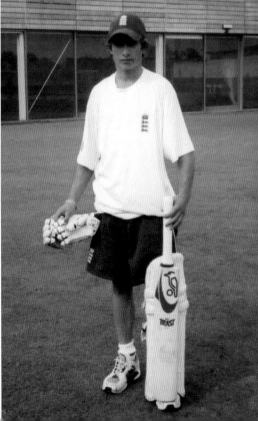

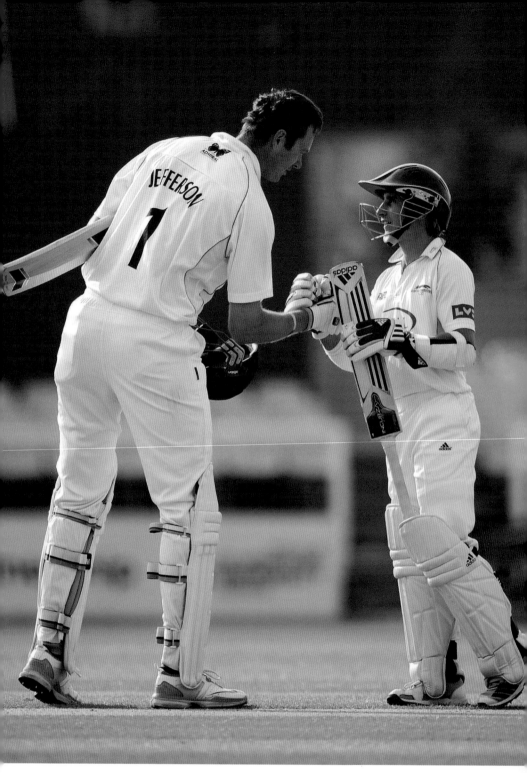

Batting with my good friend, Will Jefferson, during my time at Leicestershire CCC. Some great memories from my time there. (Getty Images)

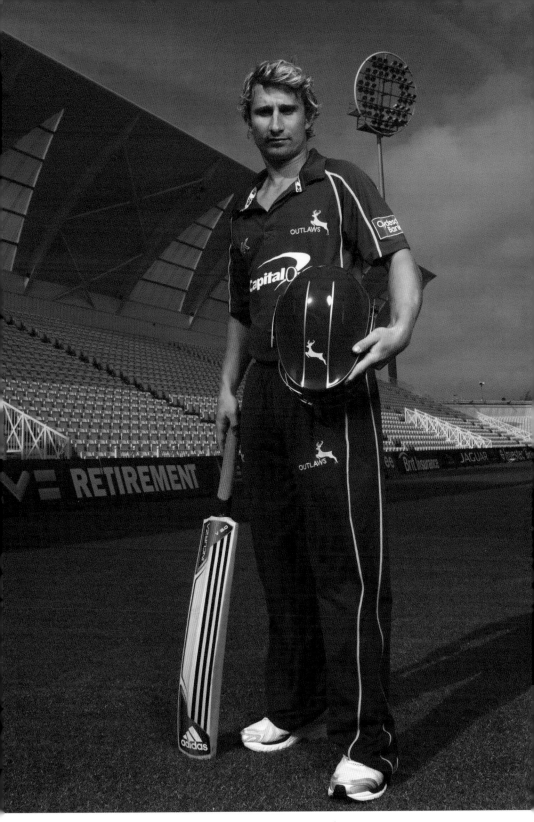

Me and my highlights at our first press day with Nottinghamshire CCC. (PA Images)

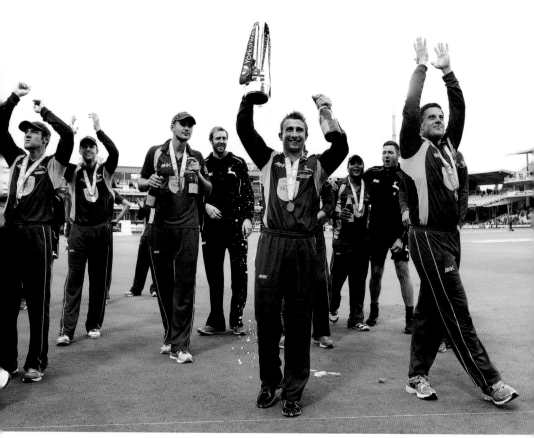

Celebrating winning the YB Pro 40 Final at Lords in 2013 with Nottinghamshire CCC.
(Getty Images)

Driving at Trent Bridge! A place where I developed enormously as a player and person. (PA Images)

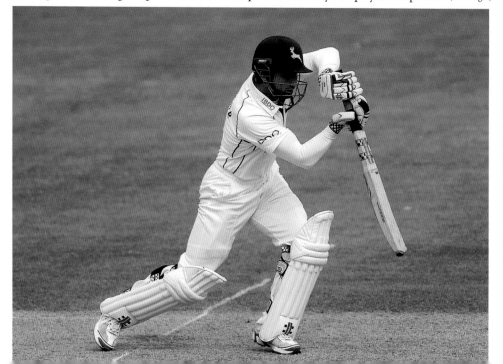

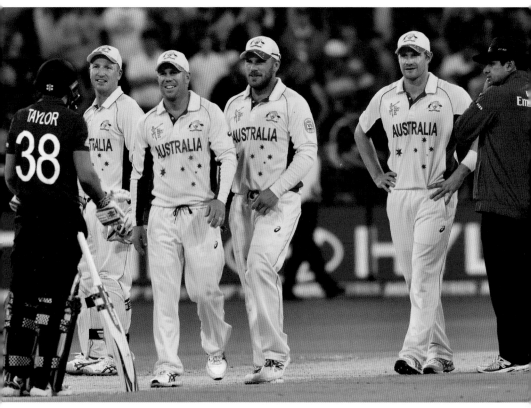

Just a friendly conversation with a lovely bunch of lads... The 2015 World Cup - Australia vs England, MCG. (Getty Images)

A sweep shot on my way to a century in the warm up game against 'South Africa A' before the ODI series. (Getty Images)

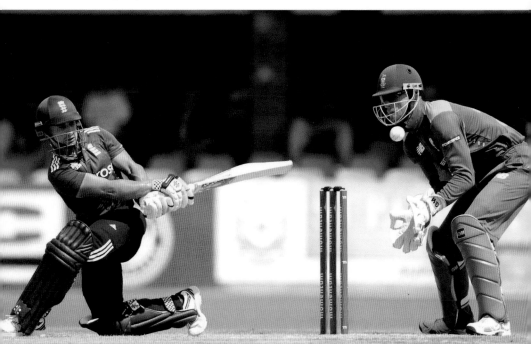

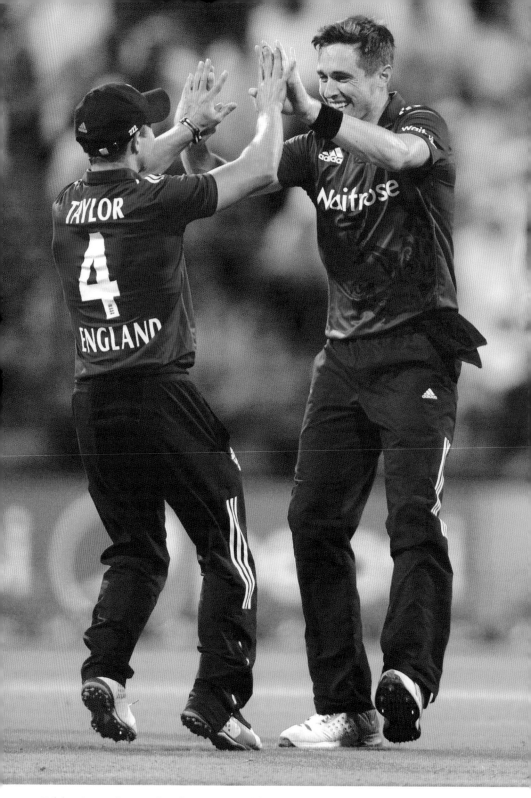
Celebrating with one of my best mates in life and cricket, Chris Woakes. (Getty Images)

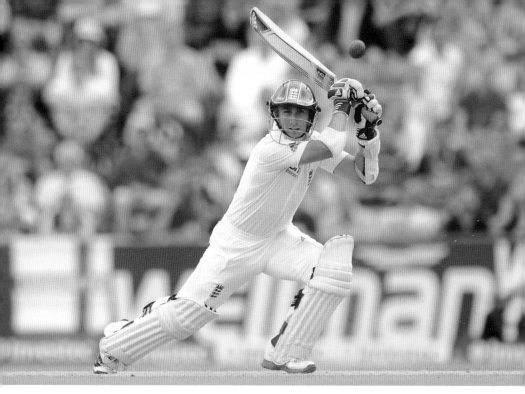

Batting during my test debut in 2012 at Headingley. (PA Images)

Rooty and I walking off at the Wanderers after celebrating knocking off the winning runs. (Getty Images)

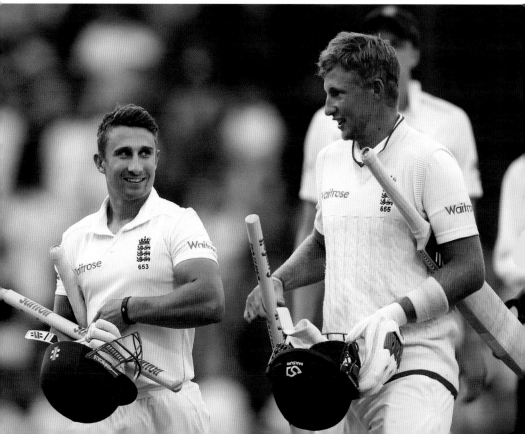

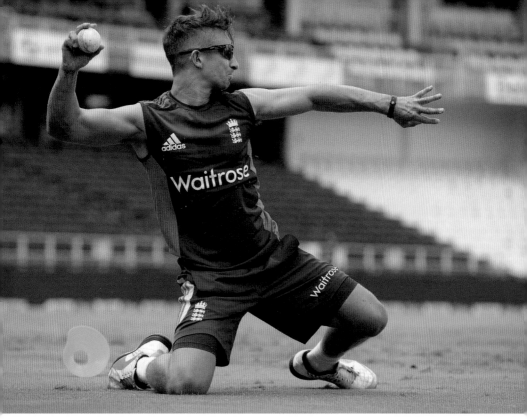

Fielding practice at the Wanderers, Johannesburg, before the 3rd Test Match in the 2015/2016 series. I prided myself on the quality of my fielding. (Getty Images)

My personal favourite: the Wanderers crowd during the Test Match in the 2015/16 series vs South Africa. (Getty Images)

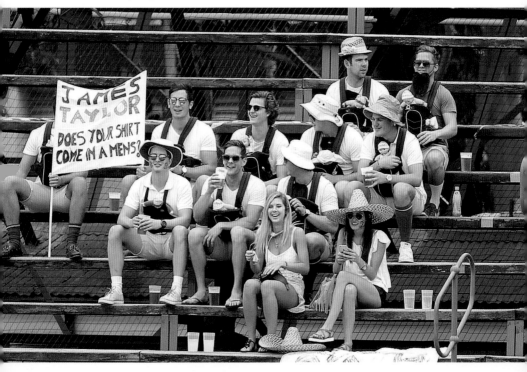

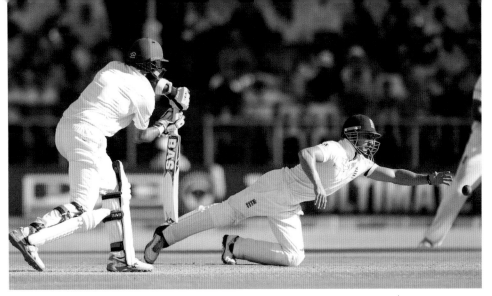

Short leg duty in Cape Town. A position I thrived in. (Getty Images)

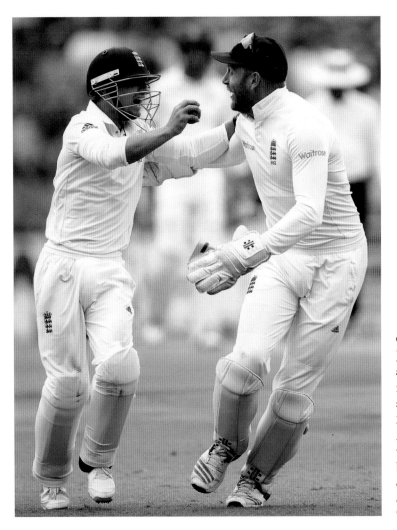

Celebrating with Jonny Bairstow after one of my catches at short leg in the 2015/16 South Africa series. It was one of the best feelings I've ever had on a cricket field. (Getty Images)

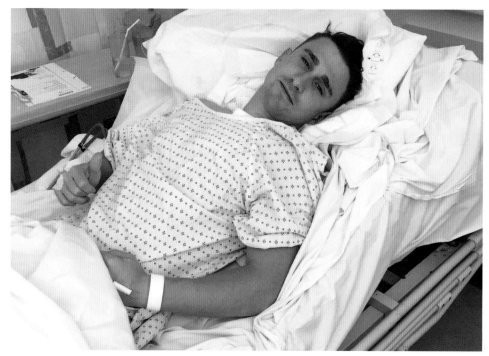

Having just come around from heart surgery in June 2016, I was delirious from anaesthetic and knew I had a mountain to climb.

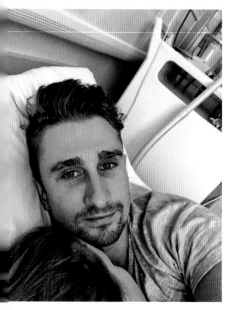

Always by my side: Jose finally managing to sleep in hospital.

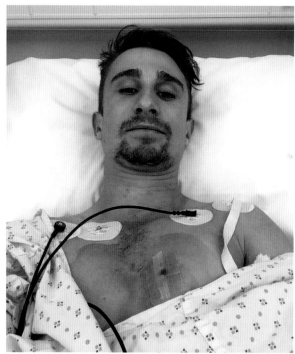

In hospital after having a minor procedure to fit a heart recording device in my chest. Surgery made a terrible mess of my chest hair!

A moment of contemplation amid the constant fear of what they might say next, as the nurse carries out an hourly check.

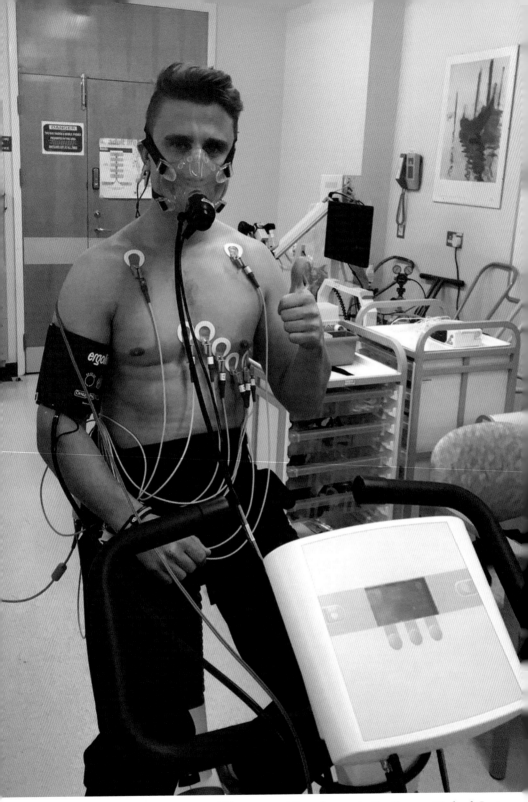

Never thought an exercise test would be so scary! Exercise test in the Queens Medical Centre Hospital, Nottingham.

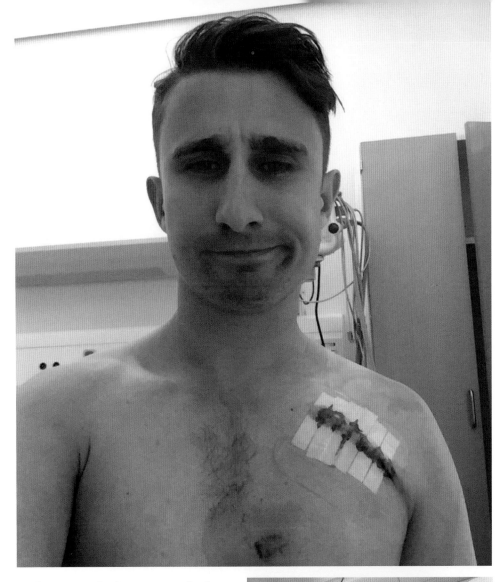

Ouch! Having a look at my scars for the first time since the operation in June 2016.

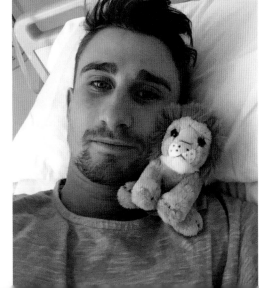

Me and the lion that Luke's kids, Albie and Amelie, gave me.

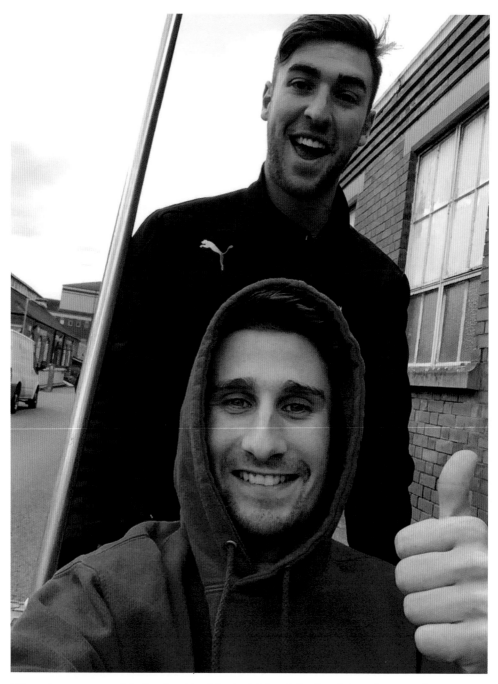

When the cats away... My first breath of fresh air! Sam Wood and I sneaking out for some fresh air for the first time in seven days while Jose left the hospital, haha!

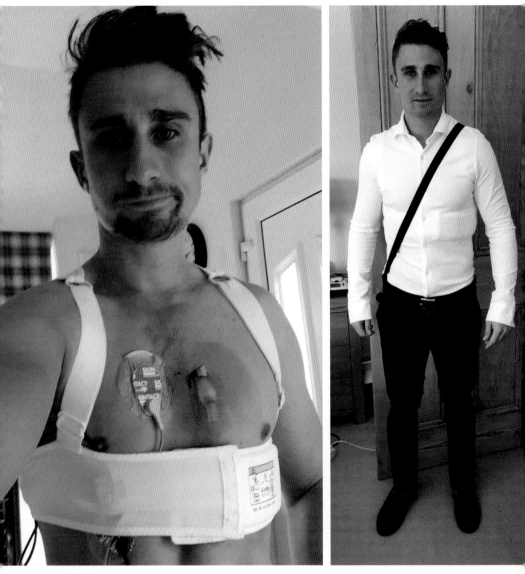

Baggage: getting home with things strapped all over my chest.

What life vest?

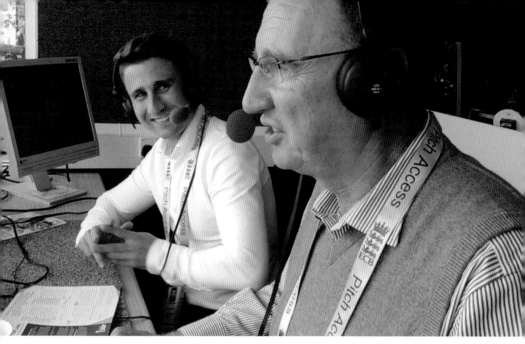

Every cloud... Working with legends while commentating with Test Match Special.

The joys of commentary mean the best views in the house (Optus Stadium in Perth, Australia).

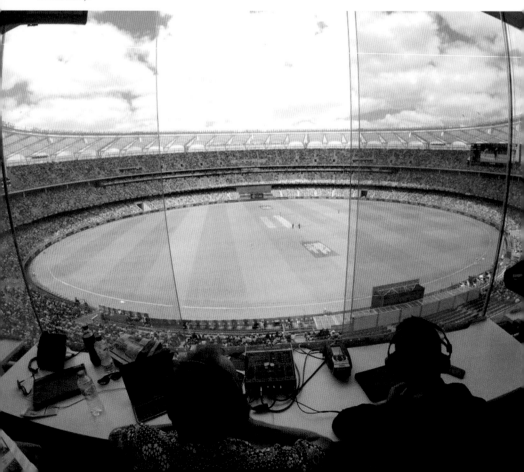

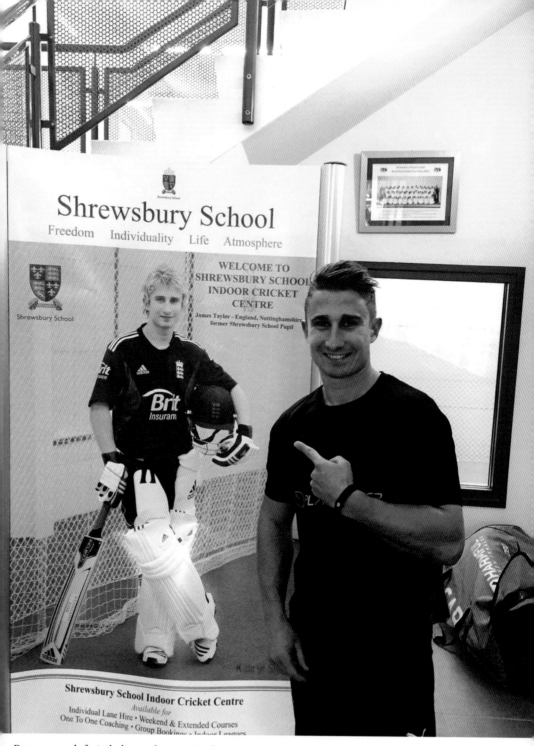

Better tan, definitely better haircut! Indoor school at Shrewsbury school.

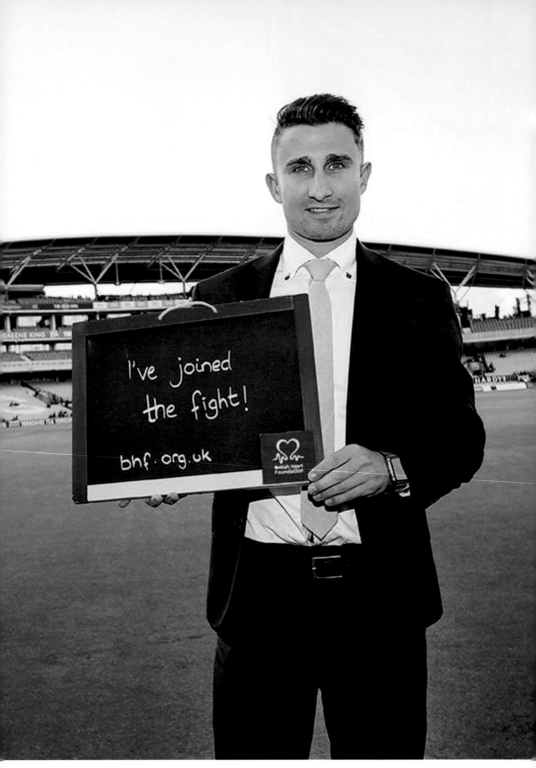

It has been an absolute honour to work as a British Heart Foundation Ambassador.

The moment after
Jose said yes!

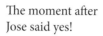

Flying! Our first dance.

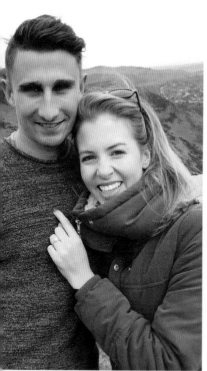

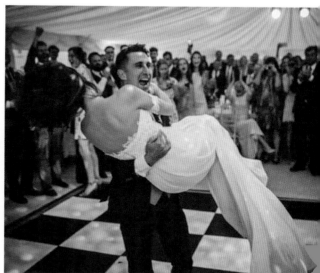

I know, I know; I'm the lucky one.

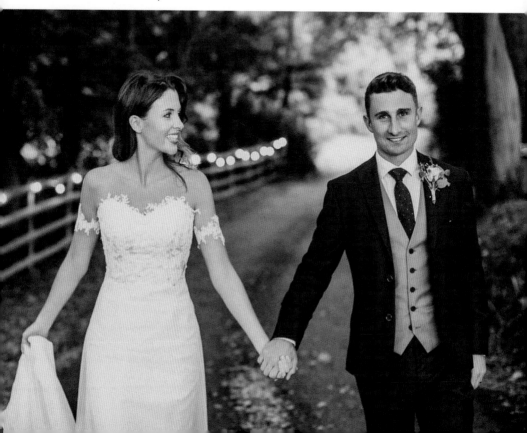

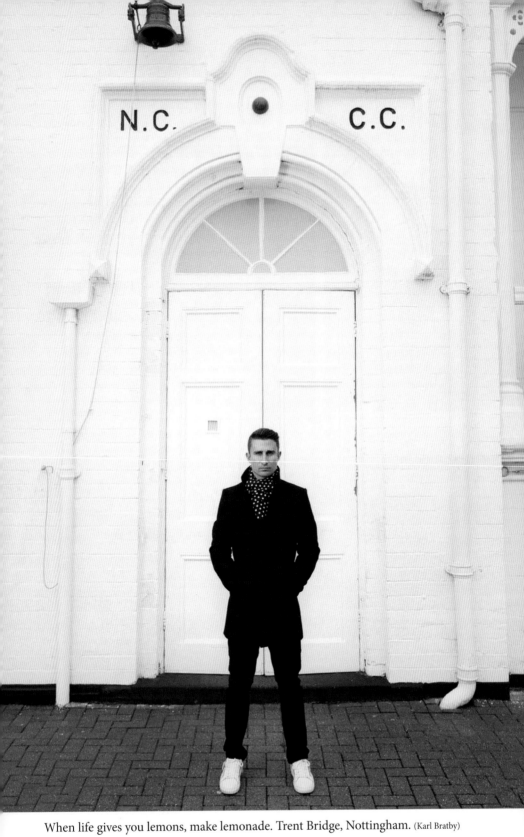

When life gives you lemons, make lemonade. Trent Bridge, Nottingham. (Karl Bratby)

helpless. All Jose could do was hold me. She wanted me to know I wasn't alone – that she was close enough to experience the shock too. 'If it shocks you, Jim, I'm here. Just let it kick in.'

It's so hard at moments like that to stay still, just waiting. Waiting for something so drastic. I got up and began pacing around. I was shaking my head. 'It's fucked, Jose.' I kept saying it over and over. And that's how fatalistic those moments feel. How close to the edge you really are. There's no turning back. If it wants to take you over the side, that's exactly what it will do. But that doesn't mean you won't try anything, however pointless, to stop it – sitting down, standing up, pacing around a small room. It's a physical agitation; you have no choice but to go along with it.

Then, out of nowhere, relief. Calmness was returning, my breathing coming back to normal. I sat, and then lay down on the bed. My eyes were shut and I was no longer stressed. I started swallowing normally again. When my heart's not good I swallow like I've got a sore throat.

'What's happening now, my love?' Jose asked me.

'I think it's all right,' I said quietly. 'Yes, I think it's all right now.'

We came down in the morning and Amie and Chris were cooking us scrambled egg. 'Sleep well?' they asked.

'Yeah,' I replied, 'but my heart was a bit dicky.' I've got a knack for understatement.

Bearing in mind that these kinds of occurrences, at one extreme or another, weren't uncommon, the thought of a night apart wasn't easy for either of us. Every summer, Jose and Libby would take their mum to Cornwall for a treat. It was just for a few days and I was confident I'd be fine. That's exactly what I told Jose. But that's not to say I could ever guarantee my heart wouldn't have other ideas in the middle of the night. On the other hand, I knew Jose would be there for me on the other end of the line day or night. I also knew this was another stage towards something resembling normality. We couldn't do this forever. Jose needed to go back to work, we both needed to understand what it was to be away from each other, and we needed to trust in John Walsh's words: 'The defib is there so you can have a normal life.'

As a professional cricketer I had spent countless nights, weeks, months even, away from Jose. That was my life, and, staying in the game in some capacity, it will likely be my future too. I couldn't hide away from stepping stones like this. I couldn't always fear I was going to be carried away in a flood.

The Cornwall test turned out fine. We both passed. But as I lay alone in bed, the first time since that fateful day in Cambridge, it did undoubtedly feel strange, disconcerting, to know that Jose was no longer by my side. Whenever I'd felt the slightest twinge, or anything out of the ordinary, I was so used to telling her, to her listening and helping. Now, for the first time, I couldn't roll over and ask, 'Can we just talk?'

Little by little, though, we were moving forward. Everything that was put in front of us we would somehow overcome. But there was one barrier that was like a canyon in the road. That whole situation at Leicester when my defib had gone off had come from the unknown – the fact I didn't know what my life was going to look like or where my income was going to come from. That might sound odd for an international sportsman, but when the ARVC finally struck that day in Cambridge, it did more than leave me a shell of my former self; it revealed a void of communication that truly terrified me.

Chapter 7

Debut

I was twenty-one years old, standing in front of the panel on *Dragons' Den*. Except instead of Peter Jones, Duncan Bannatyne, James Caan and Deborah Meaden, here I had Geoff Miller, James Whitaker, David Parsons and Graham Thorpe. This array of mildly intimidating selectors and coaches wanted me to sell something to them. Not the latest gadget to save vital minutes in the kitchen – they wanted me to sell myself as a cricketer. You'd be right in thinking the England Performance Programme could occasionally be a weird and wonderful place.

Bizarre as this setup might seem, I quite enjoyed it. It gave me a chance to say why I rated myself. The panel would ask questions and then I'd go back at them. It was a character assessment, pure and simple, but while that kind of thing can be intimidating, causing a player to clam up, the *Dragons' Den* theme was clever in that it created an atmosphere of honesty with the edges smoothed off. The trick was in sounding confident rather than arrogant. Belief in yourself had to come from a place of truth or you'd be found out. When it came to my future I was just hoping that none of them were thinking 'I'm out!'

Dragons' Den was a breeze compared to our next task. With the help of Manchester Fire Service we found ourselves crawling into a claustrophobic training chamber filled with smoke. It was all about creating pressure. If you can't deal with the unknown, can't work as a team, then you can forget making it as an international cricketer – or a fireman.

At this time I was buzzing in and around the England squad. In 2010, also with the England Performance Programme, I had shadowed England's successful Ashes tour, always with a little thought in the back of my mind – 'you never know'. In reality, the performance squad is all about reaching the next stage, which is the Lions, but being so close to the full England squad I couldn't help but wonder. A couple of injuries and who knows?

I loved Australia. Not only did the pitches suit me – bit of pace, bit of bounce – but the active lifestyle was incredible. It's an amazing place to be if you're young and energetic. I'm envious of those who grow up there.

Jonny Bairstow and I shared on that trip. Based in Brisbane and Perth, we had a simple living arrangement: he did the cooking, I sometimes did the cleaning. We roomed together with the Lions for the next three years and got very close, sharing similar characteristics. Jonny is laid back and very easy going, and neither of us ever felt like we had to impress each other, which happens more than you might think in a sporting environment. With big egos and even bigger personalities, everybody is always trying to get one up on each other. When you're younger, and forced into close confinement with people you don't know so well, it's easy to feel you have to be something you're not. Jonny and I were never like that. We were always very comfortable together. We could just be ourselves with each other.

That was quite some winter. After Australia, the Lions headed to the West Indies to play in a four day competition. I really performed over there, making 190 in Barbados. It was a great time, a good standard of cricket, and when my form continued into the new domestic season I knew I had to be knocking on the door of the full England side – if not the Test team then certainly in one day internationals.

That chance finally came when I was called up for a one-off game against Ireland in Dublin. It wasn't England's best side. It was the middle of the international summer, a number of players had been rested, and I was well aware that I was in the team because certain others had been left out. But none of that was my doing. For me, it was an opportunity to make a statement. That's how calmly and deliberately I saw it. There was no big fanfare about my call-up, not in my head anyway. For me, this was something that needed to happen – the next step. It didn't come as a surprise because I believed I should already be in the side by then anyway.

As I pulled back my hotel curtains to reveal the Irish capital that morning, I was met with a chilly grey drizzle. It was a truly horrible day. 'Typical,' I thought, 'it's going to get called off.' In the end, though, the game did get under way. As I sat in the pavilion waiting to bat, I felt the most nervous I would ever be as an international cricketer. Even though it was a lesser side, it was still my England debut. Yes, the weather was rubbish and the wicket wasn't great, but if ever I was going to score runs in international cricket then this was my chance. As I reached the middle, my nerves were tingling. I didn't freeze but I was used to knowing exactly what to do. And at that moment, I didn't. I knew all eyes were on me, the attention and the cameras, which I grew to love, but on that occasion it didn't click for me. Mentally, I was investing too much in the innings and it had confused me. I had lost the clarity of how I wanted to play. Eight balls in, having scored a single, I pulled fast bowler Boyd Rankin straight up in the air and was caught. It was frustrating, a way I would never usually get out. Nerves played a role in that shot. I was out of my comfort zone.

Another reason I hated getting out, in any game, was sitting back in the pavilion watching other people scoring my runs, especially when they were easy runs to be had. Ireland was a big opportunity for me, on a big international stage, to get some runs on the board. Ideally, I'd have taken that chance. Instead I came away feeling irritated and annoyed. At that point, everything felt pretty bleak, but over time I realised I had learnt a lot. I understood it was vital to keep a clear mind, take the knowledge I had accrued over a long time, and employ it. That was the positive I could take from the experience, that I wouldn't make the same mistake again.

That same summer I received a phone call from England's head of selectors confirming I'd been picked again for the Lions. 'Brilliant,' I thought. Then came his other announcement: 'You're going to be captain.' He paused. 'Do you want to be captain?'

I wasn't sure to be honest. I knew how hard being a captain was, especially at such a young age and with much more experienced lads around me. But you can't just turn down being captain of the England Lions. I wasn't going to say no, even though I did have some doubts. Aged twenty and captain of the Lions? It doesn't look too bad on the CV, does it? So while a little man on one shoulder was shouting 'Say no – you don't need it', his mate on the other shoulder was being a little more rational: 'England Lions captain – if you say no to that it's going to be a massive mark against your name.' He was right. Turn down something like that and it changes people's perception of your character. Selectors put you in these situations because they want you to learn. On the pitch they want you to accrue tactical nous and experience. Off it they want to make you think about the subtleties of handling different types of players.

It wasn't that I disliked captaincy per se. There was a gene in my body that meant I always had to be doing something – I wasn't one for downtime – and so being busy and organising was right up my street. It was more that I didn't want the hassle of delivering a team talk, especially to guys who were often a lot older than me and had played much more cricket. Talking in front of your peers is a difficult thing at any age, but even more so when the age gap is pronounced and you're at the lower end. Even though I'd achieved just as much, if not more, as the players in front of me, I was a reluctant captain, confident in myself but also a little introverted, so not naturally geared up for it. But, for my own progression, I had to bash on and do it.

Not being hugely vociferous off the pitch, I always thought it was easier for me to be a captain who led from the front, who set a good example.

That generally worked as I never really had a nightmare period with form. That's not to say I was always on form, but even when I wasn't I still usually managed to score runs. When I was captain of England Lions in Bangladesh and Sri Lanka in early 2012, however, I was going through a bit of a drought. Both the form and the runs had disappeared. On an England Lions tour everyone gets picked on merit, and if they're not performing they get dropped. Everyone, that was, except me. I wasn't being dropped because I was captain. When some lads should have been in the team but weren't, and they were quite vocal lads, sometimes significantly older, and I was keeping my place because I was the captain, that was a tough place to be. I wanted to get dropped, but I wasn't going to drop myself. I was waiting for the selectors to make the decision. It would have been a relief if they had.

Thankfully, my form returned. Against the West Indies next summer, I took 118 off their full bowling attack. I was very comfortable and I thought it might have got me noticed in terms of selection for the full Test series. However, while England had been having a few problems finding stability at number six, it seemed I was never the front cab on the rank. Jonny Bairstow, Eoin Morgan and Matt Prior had all filled, and consequently vacated, the role.

When the next incumbent, Ravi Bopara, withdrew from the squad to face South Africa, England's opposition in the second half of the season, however, my name began to be mentioned in earnest, not exactly hindered by me cracking 163 not out against Sussex at Trent Bridge. Soon after, I got a call from Geoff Miller. When the second Test at Headingley came round, I'd be England's fifth number six of the year.

Jubilation doesn't quite describe how it felt to receive that call-up. All the hard work, right from Maidwell onwards, had been leading to this point. That's not to say it wasn't daunting, aged twenty-two, to walk into a dressing room of that stature. Stuart Broad and Graeme Swann made it easier because I'd played with them at Nottinghamshire, but in an England dressing room there are always going to be others you don't know so well with big reputations and – who knows? – big egos. Certainly, as the new boy, a plum position in the changing room wasn't going to come my way. Some of the more senior boys had got there before me and I ended up in a rather less favourable spot tucked away down the side. Matt Prior, though, was amazing. He recognised what it was to be the newcomer and straight away took me under his wing. I got on well with Matt and went out with him, Jimmy and Broady the night before the game. Somewhat foolishly, I tried to go drink for drink with them during the meal. Three or four pints was always enough for me to feel it the next day and sure enough, with South Africa batting first, as I walked out on to the field on my Test debut, I duly noted the telltale signs – dry mouth, bit tired. I'd had a couple more than I needed to. How had I managed that? As it turned out, I had time to recover. South Africa batted for the best part of the first two days, amassing 419. They say as a debutant it's better to have a day in the field, but that doesn't stop the nerves. I was fielding at point and I honestly had no idea where the ball might end up the first time I fizzed it back to the keeper.

With a few rain breaks it was afternoon on day three when Ian Bell was out cheaply. Then there was that familiar flurry of activity – grabbing the gear, checking I'd got everything, people wishing me luck. I always liked to build up a bit of momentum, get my energy levels up, by running down the stairs on to the field. This time I did the same, just happy to stay on my feet as the adrenalin and nerves kicked in. The difference between this Test match and the one day game in Ireland was that now I was prepared. On the way to the middle I knew I needed to compose myself and gather my thoughts. I was thinking about how their great all-rounder Jacques Kallis would be wanting to get me out. I wanted to think ahead, to make sure I understood their mindset before they applied it. When I arrived at the crease, I wanted to be 100 per cent mentally prepared.

Stepping out on to the Headingley turf, I wondered what sort of reception I was going to receive. I shouldn't have worried. The cheers of the crowd were all around me. People clapped, one or two even got to their feet. They appreciated I was an England player on debut and wanted to support and encourage me. Among them were my mum and dad, to the left of the pavilion – I knew exactly where they were from when I was fielding. There was also, I think, a definite acknowledgment of my height, especially the juxtaposition between my 5ft 7ins and the 6ft 4ins Kevin Pietersen who I joined at the wicket.

I touched gloves with Kev. He didn't give me much. 'Enjoy it,' he told me. 'Do your thing.' I didn't really know KP other than as a running joke at Nottinghamshire, where he'd played a few years previously, an association that ended somewhat acrimoniously when then captain Jason Gallian threw his kit off the balcony on the last day of the season. Whenever KP's name was mentioned in the Nottinghamshire dressing room, everybody would snigger and laugh. Mick Newell, who was at the club at the time of KP's contract, obviously wasn't a massive fan because of the turmoil his presence had caused. I try not to have preconceived ideas about people and so always intended on giving KP a chance. But the early encounters hadn't been good.

When England played Sri Lanka the previous summer, I'd been called up to have a net – a chance for the coaches to see what I was about. I had a session with Graham Gooch and KP was having a net at the same time.

'Hi KP,' I said, 'how are you doing?'

'What are you doing here?' Nothing else, just that.

'I'm just here having a net with Goochy.'

He didn't say anything else and walked off.

The same thing happened at a training session with the England lads. Everyone else came up to me – 'How are you doing, Titch?' KP ignored me. He said nothing. It was bizarre. Whether he was trying to intimidate me and be the big man, or it was him feeling threatened by me, I don't know. But this was before I'd even met him properly or shared a dressing room. He didn't know me from a bar of soap but that was how he chose to be. They say 'never meet your heroes', and if ever there was a classic case, KP was it. I loved the way he played. One of my goals was to play alongside him. But on both occasions I came away thinking, 'What a twat'.

Right now, though, here in the middle at Headingley, I was more concerned with my own ability, my own character. I really felt this was a moment I deserved. At the same time, I knew I owed everything to some key individuals. This was a time for me, yes, but it was as much for the people who had helped to get me here. That thought gave me confidence. It reminded me how ready I was, and at that moment I just wanted to show off in front of a big crowd and reveal what I could do. I had always had my doubters; now was the time to shut them up, to show on the biggest stage what I was about.

Of course, there were the routines to get out of the way first, such as taking my guard, and then doing it again, before we were off. The South Africans must have been thinking, 'Who is this little guy? What is he doing?'

I played at a wide one first up, which I probably shouldn't have done, but any nerves were settled when I got off the mark with a textbook off drive four from the spinner Imran Tahir. That was pretty much my plan for that whole innings: be patient against the seamers if I needed to and be more attacking against the spinners.

We made it through to tea, and then, twenty minutes later, as me and KP walked back outside, the first thing I noticed was the crowd laughing – the size difference was even more obvious close up. I had a little chuckle inside. It helped calm me down because going back out after tea you're always a bit nervy.

I batted fairly cautiously as we built a partnership, reflecting the position of the game, but KP was having none of that. He provided an amazing display of hitting at the other end, awesome stroke play of a kind that only he was capable. As the other batsman, it's not like you can stand and stare dumbstruck and say 'Oh my God!', but make no mistake, I was enjoying watching. It was a proper fireworks display, to the extent that a little bit of me was thinking, 'What are you doing, mate? You don't need to be doing this. We need to keep our heads down and keep batting!' But he was just whacking them, playing the innings of his life. Any normal person would never have batted like that because it was totally the wrong way to play in that situation. But this was KP – he did things as he wanted to do them, and ultimately he succeeded.

Contrary to the sheer wizardry of KP's flashing bat, his conversation in the middle wasn't quite so tantalising. As the partnership progressed, he didn't talk down to me but was super arrogant. Facing Tahir, KP sauntered down the wicket. 'I'm just debating how far to hit this next one,' he said. We put on a 147 partnership, which gave the initiative back to England, but I don't think he really considered me part of it. A few days later I heard that, during the innings, he allegedly commented that I wasn't going to be on the highlights that night.

His low opinion of me extended into the dressing room. That same day, he apparently slagged me off to other players for not being good enough and batting too slow. At the time I didn't know anything about it. I was just interested in keeping my head down and getting on with my first Test. The game ended with England facing a fourth innings run chase. I was desperate to bat and it's one of the biggest regrets of my career that I never shouted up to say I wanted to go in. I wasn't in a position to do that – no player is – but nevertheless I wish I'd had that opportunity. I had nothing to lose and only everything to gain in terms of making a statement. In the end, the run chase was aborted and the game petered out into a draw, although not before Matt Prior had been run out by Jonathan Trott. On arrival back in the dressing room, Matt kicked a box that was holding open the door. He thought it was empty. In fact, it contained about a hundred match programmes. He bust his big toe. Trying not to laugh wasn't easy.

The game might have ended but the pantomime was about to start. KP was at the press conference, we thought to give his thoughts on one of the finest centuries of even his glittering career. Instead he used it to deliver an almighty whine about how tough it was for him as an England cricketer and how the next Test at Lord's could be his last. 'It's not easy being me in this dressing-room,' he told the assembled throng.

I was with Broady, Jimmy and Matt when his outburst appeared on the television. My instant reaction was I couldn't believe what I was seeing. 'Oh my God – what is he doing?' – and it was a reaction shared by everyone else. That press conference should have been all about KP scoring one of the greatest knocks of all time. Instead it was all 'Look at me, feel sorry for me.' It was just awful, exactly what England didn't need. So, so public. The state of our dressing room, as seen through one person's eyes, had just been broadcast to millions. It transpired that KP thought a spoof Twitter account in his name was being operated from within the dressing room, or with the blessing of certain players, but whatever the rights and wrongs of KP's position, it's an absolute given in any team that what happens in the dressing room stays in the dressing room. Why would you want to air your dirty laundry in public? He clearly felt empowered by the fact he'd scored those runs, but his comments were never going to paint him in a great light. After all, there was one very obvious question that people were bound to ask: 'Why are they doing this to you, Kevin? There must be a reason.'

It was hard to take in. Playing for England had been my absolute dream. Now here I was on my Test debut, but when the game came to an end, rather than looking back on a job well done, my overriding thoughts were utter disbelief as to how Kevin had behaved in that press conference. The story of that Test should have been him playing one of the great innings. For me it was the subplot of putting on 150 with him. Instead it turned into this horrendous soap opera of his own making. Put simply, I found his antics embarrassing.

The first I heard that KP had been saying things about me was a few days later when Rhian Evans, the ECB media manager, rang me. I was driving when I saw her name come up on the dashboard.

'Hi Titch, are you all right?'

I was imagining it was just a routine call about a press interview. I was wrong. 'I just thought I'd let you know there's going to be an article coming out claiming KP had a go at you when he came off the pitch.'

'Oh, it's all right,' I said. 'It'll just be the media. They'll have made it up.'

I put the phone down and genuinely didn't think anything of it. I didn't even read the story, I was that unbothered about it. Even if there was something in it, I didn't care because I didn't respect KP due to the way he'd behaved around me. The fact I didn't seek out or read the piece illustrates where I was when it came to Kevin Pietersen. It was inevitable though that I'd find out what he'd been up to. Essentially, even before the game had even started, he was telling the coaches and other players I shouldn't be in the team, and then that continued during the game itself, despite the fact that my support at the other end had allowed him to play one of the greatest knocks of his career. It explained his attitude prior to the game. While others were welcoming me, helping me settle in, Kev was giving me nothing. Before the game, a load of new bats arrived for me at the ground from my sponsor Adidas. They were top quality, the best I'd ever had. In fact, they would be some of the better bats in the dressing room. Kevin was also sponsored by Adidas. He looked at them and gave them back to me. He said nothing. He gave me nothing, full stop.

Kevin admits his opinion of me in his book. 'His dad was a jockey and James is built for the same gig.' Classy. He admits even as he was driving to the game that he rang the England coach Andy Flower and asked, 'How on earth have you picked Taylor?'

He justifies this opinion by stating, 'The poor guy has never been seen again … so I was wrong about Taylor, was I?' Well, yes mate, you were. And that's where I am with Kevin Pietersen and his view of me – it makes me laugh. If Andrew Strauss had said those things about me, it would have been awful. It would have really affected me, because I had so much respect for him. Kevin Pietersen? I couldn't care less because I don't respect him. Kevin is a big fish and what came out of his mouth made about as much sense.

No one in the actual England setup ever really spoke to me about what Kevin had said and done. When it came to the players, many of whom had shared a dressing room with KP for years and knew what he was like, they had one piece of advice: 'Ignore it.' I don't know who in the England dressing room had leaked Kevin's antics to the papers, but one thing was for sure, they did it because they'd had enough of him.

I'm not blind to how KP must have felt. I can see that it would be a horrible position for him to be in, to feel alone in the dressing room, but it was a position he'd brought on himself. His presence had long been divisive and had caused serious disjointedness to the side. Add in a tough series against South Africa, losing the first Test heavily, the lads being tired, and one massive ego stamping around in the middle of it all and it was a powder keg just waiting to be ignited.

The England dressing room at that time wasn't in a good place. KP at that point just didn't seem a team player. I couldn't believe what I was seeing when I first experienced being in the same team as him. I couldn't believe how he behaved or how he didn't do anything. This was someone I aspired to be like. As a kid watching the Ashes In 2005, KP was my absolute hero. I wanted to score as many runs as him, to be as good as him. And now here I was seven years on, and the scales had well and truly fallen from my eyes.

I had a perhaps naïve expectation of him doing things I'd never seen before. And yet I saw him bat in a net at Headingley and he was just slogging. There was attitude pouring out of him. It was the same on the field when the match started. I couldn't believe what he was doing. He didn't say a single word to anyone. As I stood on the Headingley turf I was thinking, 'Is this really what Test cricket is about?'

At that point I hadn't realised that my role in KP's descent into self-pity and vitriol was something more than a bit part character. It's been said that several members of the team let him know what they felt about his views on me, adding to the maelstrom of 'poor me' and bitterness already fermenting in his head, and ultimately to his words at the post-match press conference. In hindsight, I'd seen the fallout from his thought process in the middle – I don't think he'd have batted that way if he hadn't been in that frame of mind.

There were two weeks between Headingley and the final Test at Lord's. If Kev's grand public speech at Leeds seemed like a big deal, it was nothing to what he'd been doing behind the scenes. It transpired that he'd been sending text messages about Andrew Strauss to the South Africans. At that point his position in the team became totally untenable and he was dropped for the Lord's encounter, with some predicting he would never play for England again.

When it came to 'textgate', it totally rang true to me as something KP was capable of doing. He was very chummy with the South Africans. I heard that he'd been told not to speak to them so much, and then he deliberately spoke to them anyway. I found it embarrassing for an international cricketer, an England cricketer, to behave like that. I had immense respect for Andrew Strauss, and to see him treated like that was awful. Lord's would be Strauss's hundredth and final Test for England. It should have been a time of celebration for one of England's great players and captains. I really felt for him – to be embroiled in all this nonsense because of the selfishness of one man was awful.

I kept asking myself, 'Is this really Test cricket?' Well, it was for me. It was all I knew. I knew nothing else. There was so much going on other than cricket when I walked into that England changing room that the fact someone was making their debut could well have been forgotten. And yet somewhere in that mix was me, a 22-year-old lad who wanted nothing more than to lap up the joy of playing Test cricket. Well, as they say, good luck with that.

Even though he wasn't there, the KP situation totally overshadowed the next Test at Lord's. There were a lot of murmurings and rumours about outcomes and consequences – people wanting to know exactly what had happened, which is only natural. Before the match, the ECB tried to deliver some clarity by calling the players to a meeting in the Regent's Park Marriott, just around the corner from the ground, to explain the situation. KP had been left out, Jonny had come in, and we got a bit of a run through as to where the ECB stood in relation to KP and his future, or otherwise, in the England side. For my own good, I tried to put the textgate ramifications to one side. I was new to the dressing room and didn't think it was my place to get involved. I needed to get my head down and concentrate on my game.

In between Tests I went back to county cricket. In hindsight, it was a mistake. What I really needed was a rest, to replenish myself mentally and physically. Lord's was the last Test of the summer and, with a place on the India tour at stake, I knew I had to perform. I wasn't feeling the pressure as such – there was no 'this might be my last Test if I don't come up with the goods', because I knew I'd played well at Headingley. On the other hand, I might only have three innings to prove my worth and this was my second one.

Jonny's coming in meant I moved up a spot in the batting order to five. In the first innings I made it to ten before I got a quick one from Morné Morkel that found some extra bounce and I edged to Graeme Smith at first slip. Fair enough, these things happen. As a batsman you can reconcile a dismissal like that in your mind. Second time round, however, I found myself walking back to the pavilion in despair. I was batting with Jonathan Trott when he hit Dale Steyn down to the boundary at long-on. On any normal day, it would have been four, but this was the year of the London Olympics and the ball slowed as it reached an area still suffering the after-effects of Lord's hosting the archery event. Trott turned after the third run and started coming back for a fourth. I accepted the invitation, cruised towards his end, only for him to turn his back and leave me stranded yards down the pitch. Trying to run back 22 yards when Dale Steyn is stood there with the ball in his hand is never going to be easy. I couldn't believe Trott had done it to me. He'd run me out – while I was running his runs. When I got back into the changing room, I felt numb. I was so angry and disappeared into a back room to gather my thoughts. That was my opportunity to make a statement, my chance to show I could do well against a top class attack, and it had gone. I'd actually felt good at the crease. I just needed to get in and get some confidence. At lunch, Trott grabbed me.

'I'm sorry.'

Fine, but what good was that going to do? I didn't give him a lot back.

'It's all right,' I said and walked away. I was so desperately disappointed.

Before the season ended, I bumped into KP when Nottinghamshire played Surrey. He couldn't have been more chummy.

'Hi mate, how's it going? All good?'

For some reason I wasn't feeling particularly conversational.

'Yeah, all right.'

It felt like he knew he'd messed up with me and was trying to make amends. I wasn't that interested.

A few years later, I had an entertaining little Twitter exchange with him. He'd hashtagged a sporting tweet #bringbackJT. Except he wasn't talking about me. He wasn't talking about cricket even. He was talking about football. JT was John Terry. I knew that, but thought I'd jump in and quote tweet it. 'Thanks mate,' I wrote, 'always loved batting with you.' The tongue was so far in my cheek it was almost coming out the other side.

He bit back really hard. 'No mate,' he said, 'I did the batting.'

'I think you'll find they came to watch me,' I replied. 'You were too boring.'

'Nobody would come and watch you bat,' he snapped back.

My Twitter was in meltdown. Everybody loved it. Including me.

Chapter 8

Heart of the Matter

There is one thing I get asked more than anything else when people hear about the day of my attack. 'Why on earth weren't you taken straight to hospital?' Believe me, it's a question I've asked myself time after time. But I don't sit here looking to assign blame to anyone. The whole complex situation was something cricket had never experienced before and, in truth, wasn't adequately prepared for.

I was an England cricketer, on oxygen, struggling with my breathing, and telling people I was experiencing heart palpitations. Clearly, knowing what we now know, taking me to hospital would have been the right thing to do. Especially bearing in mind the best heart hospital in the UK, Papworth, is pretty much next door. In fact, when Jose rang my mum on the day of the attack, her immediate reaction was, 'He's in Cambridge. That's near Papworth.' She had a friend who suffered from ARVC and had a transplant there. She knew it was the best place in the country. But I was already on the way back to Nottingham at that point.

She couldn't believe it. 'Why on earth is he going back to Nottingham when there's Papworth right next door?' It was a fair question. Forget the fact I was an England cricketer, if anyone, whoever they are, was in a world of bother, like I was at that time, surely the thing to do is to get them straight to hospital.

At the time, that option fell by the wayside early on because everyone was working on the assumption that I probably had a virus and no one knew I possibly had an underlying heart condition. Hindsight is a beautiful thing, but the lessons learnt from my story will and have been used to put much better systems in place at the ECB and throughout county cricket. If we knew then what we know now, then my situation would have been put to bed straight away. The fact I was experiencing an issue with my heart would have been setting light bulbs flashing and alarm bells ringing from Cambridge to Lord's to Nottinghamshire and back again. Twice previously I'd had tests on my heart. Twice previously they'd shown up irregularities that needed further investigation. But neither John Alty and Nottinghamshire nor the England doctors had any idea. And neither did I. I had no idea how significant the results of those tests were. When they were never followed through and results became lost in the system, I was essentially left fighting a six-hour battle for life that should actually have lasted as long as a blue light journey to a nearby hospital.

I was nineteen when in late 2009 I had my first check-up with Cardiac Risk in the Young (CRY), a charity that works to prevent sudden death and screens players, at Loughborough. CRY had volunteered their services to the ECB in an initiative that was still very new to cricket and sport in general. The knowledge of heart issues and how they could impact on those taking part in sport was still in its infancy. This was as much a pilot scheme as anything. There was no formal screening in place in county cricket at this time because it was all so new. No one knew then how important this fairly relaxed arrangement could be to me.

I was with Leicestershire at the time of the testing, while also moving from the England U-19 setup to the England Lions. An electrocardiogram (ECG), which measures the electrical efficiency of the heart, was carried out, which was not thought to be normal, while an echocardiogram, a more advanced ultrasound procedure, suggested thickening of the right ventricular wall. Further tests were recommended and early in 2010 I went down with Mum to St George's Hospital in London. This time, while the echocardiogram was normal, there remained issues with the ECG. A more detailed MRI scan was advised but for a catalogue of reasons, it never happened.

To me, at the time, these tests were nothing out of the ordinary, a matter of routine. I had no reason to view them as anything else. They were something that needed doing, so I did them. I never thought any more of it and was told I was fine to carry on playing. Those screenings, however, revealed results that were consistent with the condition with which I was eventually diagnosed. Effectively the tests had identified a major element of what nearly killed me seven years later – I had an electrical pattern on my heart tracing that raised the suspicion of an underlying heart disorder. The test didn't show I had ARVC, but the abnormal electrical pattern should have raised concerns that I may get it.

With CRY volunteering their services there wasn't an organised system in place to coordinate results and follow-ups between themselves, counties and the ECB. I was left to sort out the MRI scan myself. I was young, touring, playing all the time. Inevitably, chasing up hospital appointments wasn't a high priority. I was a young man, who'd trained relentlessly to make myself super-fit. I'd never felt better. I just wanted to crack on – especially me, being the sort of person I was, playing sport and looking at a serious future in the game. I was getting my head down and looking to the future. I had such a busy diary. In fact, barely had the second round of tests finished than I was straight into a relentless period of cricket, starting off with a game playing for the MCC against the previous season's county champions Durham in Dubai. The result was those tests were never followed up. But I personally had taken two days out of my routine to have them done. It's not like I just ignored the whole thing. I was a willing participant.

Over those two days, the test that could have shown up the issue, were it there at that time, an MRI, wasn't done. If it had been, chances are they would have found the problem when I was nineteen or twenty. No one can say when I developed the condition, but one thing we do know is, it didn't just develop overnight in April 2016.

Next year, the ECB did want me to have a follow-up test. This was in November, and again I was travelling overseas, this time for a lengthy Lions tour of Bangladesh and Sri Lanka, and so matters drifted by. I got back to Nottinghamshire and it never happened.

It was three years later that I had the same tests with CRY as I had back in 2009/10. The ECG pattern I presented in 2014 was similar to the one I presented when tested in hospital in 2016 – a pattern that raises suspicion of ARVC. A clean echocardiogram, though – my heart was deemed 'structurally normal' – meant no follow-up MRI scan was advised to Nottinghamshire and the ECB.

Doctors tell me now that if I'd had an MRI in 2014, it would probably have shown ARVC. In both 2009/10 and 2014, had the condition been diagnosed, I would have been advised not to carry on playing cricket.

Put simply, far from what happened at Fenner's just being a random incident, something that nobody could have ever known about, it actually followed an incomplete sequence of cardiac investigations going back seven years.

I had been down to London when I was nineteen and yet the significant tests, which could well have shown exactly what was wrong, I never had. By the time I finally had the MRI in hospital in Nottingham it showed exactly what was wrong with me. By then it was too late. At no point was I ever aware how serious the consequences of not following up the tests could be. Some people will be absolutely fine. Others, however, will have exactly what I've got.

If someone had said, back in 2009/10, 'This could mean the end of your career – or, potentially, worse', then I would have acted. But it was never presented in that manner, and so I was more interested in getting on with my game. Looking back, it was early days in the whole process and so the lines of communication between the various bodies concerned – CRY, Nottinghamshire, and the ECB, and to a lesser extent Leicestershire – were underdeveloped. In the middle of it all was me, a young lad just trying to play for England and not focused on much else. I understand that dynamic now, but I did struggle to come to terms with it for some time.

Many patients fill their recovery time by doing a jigsaw. In my case, it was piecing together what had happened in my past, and how, and if, it had affected where I was now – a former international cricketer, who might well have been a dead international cricketer. It didn't take long for me to realise that clearly in the past there had been key moments and findings that should have been flagged up. That way, as soon as I mentioned my heart at Cambridge, those in charge of my care would have been able to react quickly and appropriately. I'm certain that, had they been fully aware of the facts relating to my heart history, John Alty, Nottinghamshire, and the England doctors would have taken a different course of action. Someone would have made that simple decision: 'Get him to hospital – now.' It's another reason I apportion absolutely no blame whatsoever to them for what occurred.

Even without the MRI scan, the results had flagged up that I had an enlarged heart (at the time, not realising the potential repercussions, I remember boasting about it to Jose). Yes, that's prevalent in sportspeople – chances are, I would have a big heart because I was training a lot and I was fit – but it's also, I now know, a clear signal of a potential cardio-myopathy, which is linked to sudden cardiac death. On that basis, had that knowledge been available to the physio and medical staff, the second I mentioned my heart, an ambulance would have been on its way. It has never been lost on me that for seven years every ball I faced could potentially have been my last. I was unwittingly clinging to a line of communication that wasn't yet developed to cope with the weight of my possible condition, liable to lose my grip and plunge into an abyss at any time.

For Jose, especially, there was one awful realisation that struck her more than anything – that this condition gets worse with exercise. All she could think about was the last few years I'd been full-on exercising. We went over it again and again.

'You can't put all those years of strong exercise on a heart that can't tolerate it,' she pointed out, 'and ultimately makes it worse, and accelerates the condition.'

And she was right. My condition is accelerated with activity and exercise. So being fit might have saved my life – not many people can survive six marathons in a day – but it also probably accelerated my illness. It may well be further on down the line because I carried on playing professional sport for six years after my original tests flagged up that there was something wrong. We tried, we really did, not to get angry – in my new state, conscious of keeping my heart rate low, I couldn't afford to – but it was hard.

The bottom line for me was that there were screenings, and each time I was screened something came up. And yet, at the vital moment when I needed that history to be available, nobody knew about it. Again, in hindsight, it obviously should have been a simple progression from initial complaint to hospital.

'My heart is giving me jip here.'

'OK, well on your records that's coming up as a possible issue. Papworth is just down the road. Let's get you down there straight away.'

People say I should have demanded to go to hospital, or taken the initiative and called an ambulance myself. They say I should have flagged up my previous heart tests. That doesn't in any way reflect the situation I was in. Firstly, I was being told this could well be a virus. Secondly, I had no knowledge that I might be carrying a serious heart condition. As far as I was concerned, those past tests were just matters of routine, everyone was having them. They weren't even in my head. Thirdly, my entire focus at that moment was on trying to combat and deal with how awful I was feeling. I wasn't sat at Fenner's going through my medical history with a fine toothcomb. I was simply trying to survive. I'm a cricketer, not a paramedic.

Understandably, most people thought I'd be OK financially after I retired. It would be a simple matter of the ECB and PCA filing the relevant insurance claims. The fact I was breaking my neck to earn a few quid at a prematch Q&A in Leicester would suggest different. I was on full pay in the short-term but the reason I was busting my gut that day, leading eventually to my defib going off in front of 200 people, was because I didn't know what my future looked like. I had to make that money because I had so little financial security. I was living in a time of total unknown.

In hospital, one of the few mental reassurances I had was that financially I wouldn't suffer. I was lying in bed thinking, 'OK, my career is finished, but at least I'll be looked after.' It seemed a fair assumption. I'd paid insurance all my life, was covered by policies through the PCA and the ECB, was playing Test and One Day International cricket, and was a main feature of the team. 'Well at least you'll be well covered,' people were telling me. And I agreed. That was one less weight off my mind.

Then, when I got out of hospital, and the figures started to be mentioned, I couldn't believe what I was hearing. To my mind, I was totally under-insured.

When it came to the crunch, the combined value of the PCA and the ECB's insurance policies bore no relation to the modern game. The insurance added up to little or no more than my previous year's earnings. Look at how much an international cricketer earns now compared to a quarter of a century ago. It was as if I was playing in 1990. No one had made a claim of this nature and complexity for three decades and so the policies hadn't been updated. At a time when the last thing I needed was to be annoyed or frustrated, again something major had happened that was out of my control.

It was this lack of certainty that panicked me into trying to make some money. That meant I was stressed, my defib went off, and I lost another six months of independence because I was then required to give up my driving licence. The anxiety of thinking it might happen again, of having hundreds of volts shot through my heart, meanwhile, meant no more Q&As, which would have been a decent income stream. All that, though, was secondary to the emotional toll the event had taken. I worried constantly about how bad for my health it must be to have my heart restarted, and the ongoing issues I might face.

Let me make one thing clear: my life is not about money. Those who know me will say I have never been extravagant or showy. My life is simply about enjoying being alive and sharing precious time with those around me. Cricket was a huge part of that and as someone who had always enjoyed being at the peak of physical fitness, my plan was to go on until my forties. I loved the game so much.

For anyone, no matter who they are or what they do, losing their income has serious long-term repercussions. For me it was even more serious. Take a moment to consider my medical costs for the rest of my life and the fact that I had no idea how I could earn money going forward. I didn't know what I would be able to do physically and this whole situation had been dropped on me out of nowhere. With that in mind, we were looking at policies that, while paid in full, came nowhere near to offering me much security – especially since I was being told I wouldn't be receiving a critical illness cover payout. My ARVC didn't qualify for it. I couldn't believe what I was hearing. ARVC had all but killed me. Eighty per cent of the time, it's discovered post-mortem. If that's not critical, I don't know what is. I had done pretty much everything but die, and yet I didn't qualify for the policy.

Seriously? Taking away what had happened on the day itself, my life as I knew it was over. I'd barely been able to make it to my seat in the stand at

Twickenham without it feeling like I was having a heart attack. Stair after stair after stair went straight to my heart. And they were saying I wasn't critical enough? How the hell could I not be critical? What did I have to do to qualify? The policy was worded in a way that suggested a condition such as ARVC 'does not affect normal activity'. OK, so what is 'normal activity'? Clearly it differs according to how old you are and what you do. Normal activity for a professional cricketer is playing the game – which I couldn't do anymore. Even putting my sporting life to one side, from the point my ARVC came to light, I couldn't indulge in normal activity. I couldn't even increase my pace a little while crossing a road without worrying about an attack.

I was really angry that I didn't qualify. On top of everything else I was dealing with it was just too much. But there was nothing I could do. Yes, it could be argued that I should have been aware of how far cardiomyopathy was covered in the policy, but, seriously, which cricketer in their twenties checks something like that, let alone thinks they are a candidate for that sort of heart condition? I wish I had known and done more about the insurance policies in place, but I was just trying to play cricket for England.

Jose would often break down in tears. She was angry that other people were making me angry, and I was having stress heaped on me that I didn't need, making me emotional, which I also didn't need. She was right. Through all the turmoil with my heart, the treatment, the operation, I had to deal with the trauma of trying to save some semblance of a future. These were the last emotions I needed in my head at a time when I'd already lost everything.

Bar Luke, my family, and the ECB, I was hiding it all from everybody. I did a lot of interviews where journalists would ask if cricket was looking after me, if the insurance was OK, and I'd just quietly mutter 'Yes' in an attempt to bypass the question. Journalists and the public alike assumed I was going to be looked after because I was an international cricketer and compensation would reflect long-term loss of earnings. At no stage was that the case. Instead I was dealing with what I was going through and then obscuring the aftermath to avoid a firestorm. Imagine for one moment what that felt like. My life was in turmoil because I couldn't exercise ever again. I couldn't do the job that I loved and defined who I was. And I was hiding the truth of the situation. Every time people would ask me, 'Did you know about this before? Did you have check-ups?' I'd always say something noncommittal: 'Everything seemed OK. Nothing to worry about.' I had six months of this while I had everything else to deal with on top. Nobody knew. Imagine what that was doing for me. I thought I had insured myself, as a young man playing international cricket, and yet I was staring into a black hole.

I couldn't help thinking how this could have been a very different scenario … how this could well have been a 'live' story with me dead in it. Imagine if I'd been stuck in traffic on the A14, a road that isn't exactly alien to major traffic hold-ups. Imagine that. These are fine lines. I'm getting worse and worse. What about if I'd not forgotten my keys? Instead of my mum finding me at Trent Bridge, I would have been able to let myself in and been at home on my own. Yes, Jose might have come back, but equally she might not have. I could have died alone on my sofa. I was so lucky that the ifs went my way that day. One wrong turn, one character in the story missing, and I could have been dead.

The ECB rightly decided to commission an independent report to look into the facts of what had happened to me, and why, and of course I went along with it because I wanted the facts as well. I was dealing with such a range of emotions at the time, including anger, that I found it difficult to feel warmth towards the ECB at this time. I wasn't particularly friendly towards the ECB doctor who came to see me in hospital after I had my defib fitted to ask me if I'd take part in the report. I was trying to process everything that had happened to me and it wasn't easy. I just needed time.

For me, the report involved sitting round a table in London with a doctor. I made my point of view clear: 'Why was I at risk for so long?' I wanted the doctor to understand what it was to have been a ticking time bomb, every little bit of exercise potentially pushing me one step closer to the detonator.

When the report was produced it was deemed not to be thorough enough and raised more questions than answers. So a second report was commissioned. The delay was hard. The whole matter was dragging on and on, and all the time in the middle of it I was trying to patch my life together, coming to terms with my new vulnerability, what I could do, what I couldn't, how I was going to earn money, be a dad, play with my kids in the garden.

When it was eventually agreed we could see the second report, Andrew Strauss rang Luke in advance. He said he knew when we read it we would find it difficult, basically because it assigned some responsibility to myself. It said I'd been communicated with regarding my heart and I'd not responded. But ultimately I really struggled with that finding. A 20-year-old not being as switched on as he should have been didn't seem as important as some of the other issues that came out in the report. Surely more pertinent was how a player who had been tested and had shown irregularities could simply be lost. Heart screening and the system behind it in professional cricket were not fully developed and there was no continuity in the system. There was no continuity in the system. That's not a specific dig at the ECB, it really isn't – they were at the beginning of building a system that would deal with a case like me – it was more my frustration that I was too early for that development.

It hurt. I had always wanted to play for England and now here I felt like I was in a discussion over whose responsibility it was that I nearly died. It felt like everyone was getting nervous about the situation. It was too much for me.

I would be lying if I said we didn't consider all my options, including legal ones. This wasn't something I looked on lightly or with any joy. Luke particularly cautioned on it, but I was going to be suffering badly financially as a result of what happened to me and we needed to consider everything.

At the same time, my situation was very complicated, with lots of different people and organisations involved. Trying to go to court with anyone would cost a lot of money and wasn't straightforward. Not only that, but I risked burning a hell of a lot of bridges. Who was going to be dragged into it? How was it going to be perceived by the public?

I kept hearing the argument that I hadn't taken enough responsibility for following up my initial tests. But how many youngsters chasing their dream of playing for England are trawling through their emails at that age? However, my perceived inaction was something that, in a legal sense, could come back at me.

My parents were particularly angry, and I had plenty of other people telling me it was this or that person's fault. But nothing is ever that simple.

Discussions went on for months. For a long time it seemed no one quite understood what I'd been through, how life had changed for me. It felt like it just hadn't clicked with people how close to the end I'd come, how ARVC had flipped my life upside down completely. Sadly, I didn't feel the PCA, who players rely upon to represent their interests in disputes, be it with county, country, or whoever, were really fighting my cause. It genuinely felt like it was just me, Jose, Luke and my parents fighting the fight. At a time when I needed a light at the end of the tunnel, it felt like yet another bulb going out.

In the end, I met with Andrew Strauss again in Nottingham. It was meant to be a chat, a review of the situation, but I'd had enough of the endless to and fro, the manoeuvring. At a time when I needed some sight of a road ahead, the only place talk seemed to take me was down yet another despairing cul-de-sac.

I was blunt with him. I told him how things were – how they really were, not what he'd read in the papers or heard on TV. I told him in stark, honest terms what I'd been through, what ARVC had done to me, what it had reduced me to. I told him how it had stolen my future.

'I nearly died,' I told him, 'and all the time these insurance policies weren't sufficient. And then, at a time when I've got everything else to deal with, my heart, losing my career, the fear, the stress, I've had to keep everything quiet.'

It was an outburst I'd been holding in for months. I'd hidden the truth for so long, in so many interviews.

'Don't worry,' he said. 'We'll look after you.'

'OK, but what the fuck does that mean?'

I didn't want to speak like that. I respected Strauss, always have done, always will. But I felt like I wasn't being truly listened to. I didn't go stupidly hard at him, but I was forceful. I appreciated the fact he was talking to me, and had made the trip, but it felt as if he didn't know enough about the whole situation.

The meeting ended a little acrimoniously. I wouldn't say Strauss was shocked, but equally he probably wasn't expecting it. The point was, he had seen, and heard, exactly what I was going through.

What hurt more than anything was how the whole scenario had been reduced to money. Yes, the money is important – vital; who knows what my medical costs will be in years to come? But more than that, I just wanted recognition. Nobody will ever know if playing those extra years of cricket after that initial test made my heart worse. Exercise is, after all, one of the things known to accelerate the condition. I just needed a little acceptance of that. Turn off the coolers and give me some warmth.

I wanted some initiative to come from the ECB, a move on their part that would signal a readiness to at least contemplate their role in the situation. A few weeks later, Luke and I got called to a meeting at Lord's with Tom Harrison and ECB director of operations John Carr.

'We owe you an apology,' Harrison told me. 'I'll make it public if you want me to. Our system wasn't able to cope with what happened to you.'

The relief was massive. The best pain relief I've ever had. That single word, 'sorry', meant the world to me. Up until that moment I don't think they'd realised how important it was for me to hear it. It was a hugely emotional moment for both Luke and me. I will always respect Tom's words and the manner in which he spoke to me. To go into that meeting and hear him be so positive and understanding was amazing. It meant a hell of a lot knowing not only had they taken some responsibility but they had my back. Tom identified that I had a future, and the ECB would be part of it. After the six months I'd had it felt like I'd won the World Cup. It was such a weight lifted off my shoulders. To know I had some support in the future was huge. To have had my earning potential taken away from me, with all the lingering insecurities about my future, was like dragging a weight behind me – a weight I was ill-equipped to carry with half a heart. All of a sudden, that weight had been replaced with the candyfloss of security.

That whole period had been so incredibly draining and I appreciated that the ECB had acted and brought it to an end. From that point on, it felt like we could all move forward. I'd never wanted to be in conflict with the ECB – even the thought of it made me feel ill. I wanted there to be mutual trust and respect between us, and that's the position we're now in.

Commendably, the ECB has used my case to tighten up procedures and ensure that if a situation arises with another player everyone is better placed to deal with it. It has smoothed out those potholes of communication. I hope beyond hope that if ARVC occurs in tomorrow's cricketer it will be found and diagnosed early. If that is the result of my case, then I genuinely am pleased.

But I can't also help thinking I would quite like not to have been the trailblazer in these particular circumstances.

Chapter 9

The Size of It

When the touring party for the 2012/13 winter trip to India was announced, I wasn't in it. I was gutted. India was exactly my kind of tour. I was one of the best players of spin in the country. It made no sense. It was a real kick in the teeth.

On the other hand, whilst I was disappointed, I wasn't altogether surprised. The events of the previous summer had confirmed I was far from the top of the list. Eventually, after all other options had been tried, I was picked – in the middle of a series against South Africa, who were the number one side in the world. No one will ever know, but the West Indies may have been a very different kettle of fish. Eoin Morgan got the nod and with England also selecting Nick Compton and Joe Root, both of whom had never played a Test, and Jonny Bairstow, who only had a handful of caps, my guess is they thought I was an unsure too far.

The only reason the coaches gave me for my non-selection was a technical issue on the back foot outside off stump. It ended up being a reccurring theme over the years. I bit my tongue. I hadn't been found out with my technique. In my short flirtation with Test cricket, I'd been bowled at Headingley and then didn't get the chance to bat in the second innings. At Lord's I nicked off to a good one from Morné Morkel and was run out when it wasn't my fault. Effectively, I'd had two innings to show what I could do and performed to a good standard in one of them. The Morkel dismissal at Lord's, a low catch to Graeme Smith at first slip, was the only ball they could point to. I rarely, if ever, got out that way. Had I been selected, I would have been going to India next anyway, so a Morkelesque bowler was hardly likely to come my way. Instead I'd be playing a lot of spin, which was my strength. My technique had its quirks, but I was averaging over 50 in first class cricket before that Test match.

It hurt. It really hurt. One innings, one shot, out of the total of three innings I was given to prove myself. It was bitterly disappointing. Nothing had actually gone wrong to say my technique was a problem, and to have played a part in a 150 partnership on my Test debut said everything about my temperament. This was supposed to be the era where players got a decent run in the team. James Vince got eight Tests before he made a 50. I had three innings. It was so frustrating because I knew I hadn't got to show them what I was truly capable of.

Some people have said that talk of my technique was simply to cover up an institutional bias about my height. I never saw it like that at the time, because to me my height was never a problem. Now, though, when I step out of it, and look back on exactly what happened, there could have only have been a certain number of excuses, and my height had to have been one of them. Clearly the negativity that some people felt about me, the kind of stuff KP was saying – 'He's too small to play' – had infected key individuals in and around the England setup. Some people had to have listened, otherwise how else could they have left me out for such a long period of time?

In all honesty, I never realised how small I was until I played first class cricket. At that point I found myself up against big bowlers, big lads. Also, I'd always been that size. The nickname Titch got started at prep school. 'Little Shearer' was another because I was good at football. So it wasn't any great novelty to me. And all the way through I'd shown it had no effect on my ability or strength. I had a penalty shoot-out with some older lads at Maidwell when I was eight. They were thirteen. I broke the goalkeeper's wrist when he put a hand out to make a save.

I never minded the nicknames or the mickey-taking. On tour in South Africa with England, my teammates gave me my own step at the urinal. On another occasion, they even ordered an entire box of junior kit to be sent to me in the dressing room. I opened it up and there it was – mini bat, pads – even a box! I loved it. I put it all on. I thought it was hilarious.

For others, though, it obviously mattered. Members of the press would always refer to me as 'the diminutive James Taylor', but never once did I personally ever think 'I'm too small'. Not once, genuinely. Why would I? From the start I hit the ball as hard as most, and then when I got better and stronger I hit it harder than most. I would never think of myself as small because I was always doing better than the others, and playing with older lads from a young age, being the smallest was only natural.

I knew I didn't need to prove anything to myself about my size, but I always wanted to prove to people that they were wrong to make any assumptions about me. It wasn't so much that I would get stick off the opposition; people think there's more sledging in county cricket than there actually is, and if somebody's being a dick everybody around the circuit soon gets to know it. I did get the feeling, though, that some people were underestimating me, which, thinking positively, was massively in my favour. I knew I could exploit their prejudices by staying in my bubble, sticking to my game plan, and smashing their lazy misconceptions to the fence.

I knew I was good and knew I was good enough to get to the top. After all, height, or lack of it, had never stopped other players. Sachin Tendulkar, for instance (I'm not saying I was as good as him, by the way!) – his height made him the player he was. It added to his strength because he could get into position so much more quickly. For me, it meant I could get deep into the crease. When I started out at Worcestershire, their ex-captain Tom Moody, who himself had drawn attention for being particularly tall, said to me, 'Your height is often an advantage because you can pick the ball up quicker.' He was right. As a small man, my agility also meant I had quick feet and hands. Height to me wasn't an issue. I never let it get in my way. To me it was a unique selling point, something different. I was more difficult to bowl at because I wasn't your standard batsman. What I needed to do was prove my talent to those who mattered. Perhaps what I hadn't considered was that they might also have their prejudices. It definitely got into people's psyche. There was a perception that playing to a high level was somehow more difficult for me.

Three years in the Test match wilderness beckoned. It was as if I became a full-time Lion. I seemed stuck at that level forever. I felt as if I was marooned at university and never going to graduate. I played for the Lions for six years on and off, and captained them for four. Don't get me wrong: to pull on an England jersey in whatever format is amazing, but the Lions is supposed to be a stepping stone. For me those steps had been removed. I was floundering in stagnant water.

I tried to be pragmatic about it. My mum asked me about the situation when we were chatting one day in my kitchen. 'Well, Mum,' I told her, 'I've played Test cricket for England, life as a county cricketer isn't too bad, and if I never play for England again at least I've had a chance.'

But inside I found it unfair, and I wasn't the only one. Coaches all across the country were telling me they couldn't understand why I wasn't in the England team, and that included those coaching the Lions. Dave Parsons, Graham Thorpe and Mark Ramprakash were big fans of mine. They had seen me score more runs than anyone, but unfortunately they weren't the ones with the power in their hands.

'All you can do is keep scoring runs,' they'd tell me. And that's what I did. I kept on bashing down the door only to find another barrier on the other side. I had the ability, the averages matched up, and I'd performed on the big stage. But I simply never got a chance. I'd get stuck in, play the hard cricket, but it didn't seem to matter. It never appeared to be noticed. There was a small group of people who apparently thought I couldn't play. Their opposition seemed an immovable object. I did everything they asked of me, playing as an opener on a green seamer, answering all their questions about my technique, but when it came to that progression to the Test squad it was as if it was never meant to be. The England selectors just didn't appear to like me. Height was never specifically mentioned. They never gave me a reason, full stop.

There was the occasional chink of light to get my hopes up. Ahead of the third Ashes Test in 2013, KP had a calf problem. England requested that I play for Sussex in a four day game against the tourists, which very much suggested I was next in line. I made 121 not out, but KP recovered and that was that. I was back down the motorway to play at Taunton.

It wasn't just the selectors who thought I should go back to county cricket. When I scored that hundred for Sussex against Australia, one well-respected cricket writer basically said, 'If England think this lad is ready to play then they're sorely mistaken.' That really summed up some people's perception. Who scores a ton against Australia and then gets told they've gone backwards? For some, the attention was always on what I couldn't do rather than what I could. Maybe I didn't appeal to their ideas of aesthetics by being short. My game wasn't pretty enough for some commentators. Whatever the reason, it did feel like I wasn't playing by the same rules as everyone else. The whole topic became bigger than it actually was.

The only other person who said anything to me, and didn't beat around the bush and dress it up in technical nonsense, was England coach Andy Flower. Later in that same Ashes series, a debutant Gary Ballance was picked ahead of me.

'We've picked Gary for no other reason than we think he's the right man for the job,' Flower told me, 'and he's going to score more runs than you.'

You might think I'd be upset with that. Actually, I was perfectly happy. Yes, it's brutally honest. But I'd rather have that than be given some bullshit comment about technique. I preferred the black and white of that excuse rather than someone talking absolute rubbish or not giving a reason at all – or telling me to go back to county cricket and score more runs, which I'd done every time they'd asked me.

That drawing board was becoming horribly familiar. But I had to face it, trying to make it a more positive prospect by treating it as a new challenge. I positioned it in my head that sometimes you need to take one step back to go three steps forward. That winter, I worked really hard on getting even fitter and stronger. I'd let my work ethic, and runs, do the talking. Weight of runs would, I told myself, get me back in the frame or thereabouts. Some people's motivators are records or money. Mine was always proving people wrong. That burning desire to show people what I could do, to perform and score runs, was absolutely my biggest inducement. Being an international sportsman is the best life in the world. I'd had a sniff of it, and I wanted more.

It was hard. I continued to score heavily in county cricket, as asked, and yet was never given a shot. At the same time, every time I played international opponents I scored runs. Occasionally, I'd find myself in an uncharacteristically negative frame of mind, identifying players from other counties who I considered rivals and actively wanting them to fail. Naturally, from a purely selfish point of view, if someone else isn't doing well it makes your own stock higher. I'd look around the county grounds on the internet and be willing those players who were challenging for the same position to make a low score. I remember being at a barbecue at Steve Schofield's house and staying outside to avoid an England game on TV rather than watch others take the chance that could have been mine. That's a really unhealthy place to be, but, if they're honest, most cricketers have had periods where they've done the same. I learnt as I got more experienced and older that it wasn't helping anybody, least of all me – it was only making me angrier. It was a negative mindset that sapped me, and that was the last thing I needed. My life became a lot more enjoyable when I stopped doing it. Over time I learnt to be more carefree and understood I was wasting energy on things that were out of my control. I couldn't influence what another player was doing; I could only control what I was doing. It got to a stage where if they got a hundred it didn't bother me, and equally it didn't bother me if they got a duck.

Nevertheless, these were players who I felt I was more consistent than, and yet they were the ones taking the road that I thought I should have been travelling, while I was left behind on a permanent red light. I felt that if it was a shootout between me and them, I would have had a very decent chance of winning. My county record was better than theirs. Whenever we had played together it had been the same. Generally, I'd always performed better than Jonny in teams. Rooty showed his quality from early on, but, especially in one day cricket, I scored more runs than he did. I also knew that certain people thought they were better than me because they could play shots that I couldn't. The fact is, I could play those shots, I just chose not to, which is why I was more consistent. I'm a big believer in earning the right and yet other people seemed to earn it easier. I never said anything in case I looked bitter, which would only have held me back even further. All I could do was get back on it and work hard, on my fitness and in the gym, and score runs until they had to pick me.

Eventually, I had a meeting with Graham Thorpe at Loughborough. 'Right,' he said, 'what do we need to do to get you in the England team?' We both knew I could and should have been playing. We concluded that I had a good game but we had to make it even better, keep bolting things on, like hitting over extra cover, finding the gaps consistently, being more positive earlier in my innings, and then having other options to go to as well. Thorpe and Ramprakash were big players in my progression. Thorpe's strengths as a coach matched mine; he had been strong against spin as well as on the back foot. Ramps was also brilliant, a batsman whose love of making runs was unsurpassed. He knew me because I'd made a lot of runs against Surrey and always liked the way I played, my own hunger for runs. It certainly helps if your thoughts align with your coach and they respect the way you play rather than wanting to change it. The fact that Ramps had his difficulties translating his undoubted brilliance into a Test career makes him an even better teacher. He understands the mental battle as well as the ins and outs of technique. Like so many others before him, he invested time and effort in me. I scored 242 not out for the Lions against Sri Lanka at Dambulla and again and again he walked round the boundary looking to catch my eye, gesturing to me to keep fighting. Now I'm a coach myself I seek to build that same connection with a player. Ramps informed my coaching in a positive way.

With Thorpe and Ramps I kept my game and built on it. I took it to the next level. I was still averaging 50 in one day cricket, but instead of achieving a strike rate in the high 70s, I was now doing it at 90–100. That's not easy to ignore. I was one of the leading run scorers in the country, consistently performing under pressure and against the toughest opposition. The sheer weight of runs and quality of the performances meant the selectors had to pick me, and ultimately that's what happened. I had another, slightly more successful, run-out against Ireland in Dublin before being named in the ODI squad for the tour of Sri Lanka, although even then I had to wait three matches before getting my chance. Cooky got banned for a game for England's slow over rate in the third game and a slot opened up perfectly for me at number three for the fourth match in Colombo.

I'd never been more ready – all I needed to do now was take my opportunity. I'd scored 8 off twenty-five balls and then I took a gamble. I hit the 'Fuck it!' button, as I call it. I ran at Thisara Perera, who was bowling about 85mph, and flicked him as hard as I could over midwicket for six. That got me going. It showed everybody I had the power and the intent. It also gave me the confidence I needed. It was a risk. If I'd got out in that situation after hitting 8 off twenty-odd balls it wouldn't have looked great. Instead, though, that shot was a catalyst. I played really well from that point on and was into the 60s when I got really awful cramps – not surprising, it was 40 degrees with 100 per cent humidity. From then on I started playing more shots, simply because I had to. I'd reached 90 when I knocked one up in the air, again because hanging around wasn't an option. Back in the pavilion I was suffering full body cramps. My game revolved around quick running, fast twitch fibres, and exerting a lot of energy. In Colombo, it was a combination that paid a price. I felt like I was being stabbed from the inside. I had the first twenty overs off in the field. The other lads were calling me 'Sachin', because he would often bat and then disappear for a prolonged stay in the pavilion.

A ton would have been great, but it didn't matter. I'd been given an opportunity and taken it. What a feeling that was, back in my room, so exhausted, so tired, unable to sleep because I still had that little bit of adrenalin. That's a feeling you cannot replicate other than by scoring runs.

In my wakefulness, I looked at my phone. My social media was going crazy, and again it showed I'd done something special, but to me it was just the start of something. I'd shown that in the toughest conditions, with the ball spinning sideways, I could do it – something that not many other players could.

I took that euphoria into the next game at Pallekele as Rooty and I put on 104 to win the game. It was one of the happiest times I've ever had on a cricket pitch. We both felt so comfortable that we were messing about in the middle singing cheesy pop songs. We knew each other and each other's games so well, everything seemed easy. I felt certain we'd see the chase through to the end, and Joe did go on to be 104 not out. My innings, though, stalled on 68, that sense of freedom and abandon vanishing to be replaced by an anger I'd rarely ever felt on a cricket field. In Sri Lanka, with the high temperatures and humidity, gloves get soaked very quickly. I signalled to the dressing room for some fresh ones and Ian Bell, who was twelfth man that day, brought me out a pair, only for me to discover after he'd disappeared that they too were wet. Next ball, my hands slipped on the bat and the ball top edged straight to fine leg. I was absolutely seething when I walked off, ready to give Bell a real spray, but Mark Saxby, the England masseuse, the nicest guy in the world, managed to calm me down. I'm still convinced that error cost me a century.

That series fed straight into the preparations for the 2015 World Cup taking place in Australia and New Zealand. I'd cemented myself at number three, averaging 40 and bringing some stability to the lineup that had been missing since the absence of Jonathan Trott. On the eve of our opening World Cup game, against Australia in front of 98,000 people at the Melbourne Cricket Ground, our captain Eoin Morgan took me into the physio room. 'Titch,' he said, 'can I have a word?'

My heart dropped. 'You've got to be kidding. You're going to drop me?'

'No,' he replied. 'We're going to move you from three to six.'

'You're joking me.' Throughout the whole build-up to the World Cup, all my preparation had been about batting at three, a stabilising position far removed from the blood and thunder needed lower down the order. I'd done well there, scoring 82 against India in the tri-series World Cup warm-up tournament just three weeks before. But Eoin said they needed to get Gary Ballance in the side. He could only bat at three and therefore I had to go at six – I would be more of a power hitter at six than Gary. So there I was, walking into my final net session before for the first game of the World Cup, being told I had to play in a completely different way to what I'd been doing for the previous four months. Where previously I'd been all about laying a foundation, now I was trying to whack fours and sixes. That's a big mental change to make overnight. But it summed up where the ODI team was at the time and had been for years – panic stations. It wasn't just the batters who'd been put in the mixer the day before the game. Chris Woakes had been opening the bowling all through our preparations, but then, as I stood at point, first game of the World Cup, who do I see at the top of his mark? Broady.

'What's he got the ball in his hand for? What's going on here?' Yes, Broady was opening the bowling in Test cricket, but in the one day stuff we'd been doing it completely differently.

Back at home, my dad had received a message from Jonathan Agnew, via a mutual friend. 'Tell those Taylors to get out there,' stated Aggers, 'because he will bat. You might never get to see him play at the MCG again.'

My dad got the last seat on a plane to Dubai, the last seat on a plane to Kuala Lumpur, and then hared it on to Melbourne. He found himself sat next to a kid from Shrewsbury who'd hitched across Australia for twelve hours to see me play. Also in the ground were a whole bunch of old school pals who'd made the trip as well. It's a good job I wasn't out first ball.

Any game between Australia and England at the MCG is massive, but a World Cup ODI was something else again. It was an incredible atmosphere, a phenomenal din, which just got louder and louder as Glenn Maxwell and Aaron Finch smashed us all round the park. We were 66–4 chasing 343 when I walked to the middle. At that point, Mitchell Johnson came on. He had two slips, a gulley, and a short leg – in a one day game.

I was really nervous as Johnson ran in. 'Trust your technique,' I told myself. 'Trust yourself.'

Inside I knew my technique would get me out of trouble. It was inbuilt through thousands and thousands of deliveries faced. It was just going to react. And that's exactly what happened. That technique wasn't always the prettiest, but it did a job. It was a coping mechanism that allowed me to build an innings in even the harshest of circumstances.

Straight away the Aussies were abusing me. They were calling me a jockey, and 'Brad Haddin's son', who was three at the time. I had a really slow start and they kept shouting 'Take your pillow off your bat'. It took me a couple of overs to work out what they meant – that I was blunting it, not hitting the ball hard. I knew I had to soak this nonsense up. Wickets were going down and I just had to get through it. When I then got into gear, hitting Mitch Marsh and Mitchell Starc for sixes, they shut up pretty quickly.

'Come on, lads,' I was thinking. 'If you're going to start, you might as well keep going. You can't just shut up now.' Those thoughts showed the adrenalin was well and truly running.

As I passed 50, Johnson was still having the occasional chunter, abusing me about my Perth connections – a place I'd trained and played at a few times. I told him to shut up and just carried on as usual with my business.

I was well in and from then on I hit the Aussie bowlers round the ground. The constant loss of wickets had made it a virtually impossible task but when Chris Woakes stuck around, in my head I thought, 'We can still win this.' I knew if I was there at the end we had a chance. In any situation of that kind I would always think, 'How good am I going to look if I do this?' I would always turn those pressure situations round.

Once Chris went that chance had gone, but I continued to have the best fun – nothing feels better than whacking the Aussies. I soaked up the whole occasion. Usually, you're in your own space so you don't notice the peripheral stuff that goes on at grounds, but this time I consciously took it in. I looked at the people in the bars, took in the atmosphere in the stands – I was living my absolute dream, centre stage showing off in front of a sell-out at the MCG. It is absolute class to be involved in a game like that. Sometimes, like at Headingley, the only time you're really aware of the crowd is when you're heading out to bat, because at that point they're near, you can hear them. At the MCG, it's different; a wall of noise follows you to the square. I wanted to be able to savour that moment. I was glad I did. I'd spoken to my mum beforehand. She was right when she said 'Maybe it won't happen again'.

If the umpires hadn't made a mistake, I would have got three figures that day. My knowledge of the game was better than theirs. I'd been given out LBW and while Jimmy Anderson was out of his ground at the other end, Maxwell ran him out. I reviewed the LBW – not out. Great, on we go. But then the umpires said, 'Well, let's have a look at the run out.'

I knew that was wrong. How can you have a double play in cricket? The appeal was for my LBW. Once that had gone, that should have been the end of it. You can't then look at the run out as well. That's exactly what I was saying to the umpires, Aleem Dar and Kumar Dharmasena. The only Aussie who knew I was right was George Bailey, but he wasn't saying anything to the officials, obviously. All the rest were telling me, 'Shut up – you don't know what you're talking about.'

I was arguing back: 'I'm telling you, you cannot do that, you're wrong.'

The Aussies – and the umpires – weren't for changing their minds. So there we were; Jimmy was run out and I was left two short of a century at the MCG.

I'd been back in the pavilion about a minute when the umpires came into the dressing room to apologise. I was in the physio room with a suspected torn side so didn't see them. In truth, though, it's not so much the umpires out in the middle who bothered me. Yes, they should know the rule, but at the same time they are dealing with everything that's going on in the game – the Aussies playing hell, the noise from the crowd – and it's not easy. But what about the third umpire up there in his nice air-conditioned room? It's not that bizarre a rule. If I knew it, surely he should have.

I looked at the positives; at least I was not out, and I'd made a good score in a really tough environment. Once again, I had put my hand up and shown I could do it. Yes, there was still a little bit of 'Fuck!', but only a little bit compared to the positivity.

That World Cup, as the record books show, was like every other recent World Cup for England – a disaster. For me, I was carrying a shoulder injury that caused me a lot of anxiety. I was worried about throwing, something I was always really good at, only to now find myself with a limiter. Batting was better but my shoulder still hindered what I could do, affecting my confidence and bringing its own anxieties. I was worried about letting myself and the team down. I didn't want to be an embarrassment on such a big stage. Hiding these concerns only made my situation worse. In the big scheme of things they were nothing, but to me, playing in a World Cup, they were a lot.

So anxious was I that I played the entire tournament on three hours' sleep a night. Jose became massive in getting me through. Every night I would wake up with my heart racing, from being fast asleep to wide awake within seconds. It was always the same time on the clock – ten past three. I'd have gone to bed late, because I was concerned about not sleeping, had a couple of hours, and then woken up with the adrenalin flowing. I'd Facetime Jose and she'd be my psychologist. She'd talk me back to sleep, telling me not to worry, and then I'd have another hour or two before waking up with my eyes burning because I'd had so little sleep. It happened night after night. I was so tired and in the end talked to the team psychologist just to see if he could give me a coping mechanism that would help me relax. In the end, though, I went back to Jose. Nobody knew me, and what I needed to hear, better than her. I also had my own coping mechanism – remembering there were always a lot worse things going on in the world than me worrying about my shoulder.

'Calm it!' I'd tell myself. 'Man up!'

The occasional sleeping pill was my also blessing. When I took one of those I had the luxury of four, maybe even five hours out for the count.

My general well-being wasn't helped by the fact I'd been in Sri Lanka for seven weeks and home for just twelve days before flying out to Australia, during which time I'd contracted chronic food poisoning. Initially, I was worried it was something more serious I'd picked up in Sri Lanka, so when the doctor said it was food poisoning I was relieved.

'That's great news, doc.'

'No,' he said. 'It's severe.'

Those twelve days of supposed rest were in fact just intense awfulness. I'll spare you the details, but it still hadn't gone when I landed down under. I was batting in Canberra against the Prime Minister's XI when all of a sudden I found I couldn't focus. Everything had gone blurry. I was so dehydrated from sickness and diarrhoea that I had nothing inside me. I actually managed to get a couple of decent scores in the warm-ups, but physically I was all over the place. My guts were bad, my shoulder was in pieces, and I was dizzy – hardly ideal preparation.

Anxiety then built up from nervousness about messing up and not being the person I should be. Fielding was a big part of my game and my shoulder was compromised. To be good at something and yet to be struggling is tough.

What I did have on my side was that I wasn't the sort of player, like Jonathan Trott, for whom everything had to be perfect. Trott appeared obsessive-compulsive, but in cricket there are so many variables that perfection is unrealistic. There's a level of intensity where a player can become trapped if they're not careful. It's why, over time, I ditched my superstitions, like doing my right shoe up first, and then putting my left pad on first too. When I got more mature all those superstitions went out the window. There are so many variables in cricket, it can never be the same, and sitting in a certain place in the dressing room isn't going to change anything. For any cricketer, there always has to be acceptance that when you are playing so much and at such a high level, you can't always keep the standard as high as you'd want it to be.

It was hard not to pity those poor souls who followed us around Australia and New Zealand. Our performances were ragged, and, in the next match against the Kiwis, embarrassing. We were bowled out for 123 in thirty-three overs, so quickly in fact that we were in the field before the interval. Brendon McCullum then went into full hurricane mode, spraying our attack to all parts of the ground, to the extent that they were 112–1 off nine overs when the break came. We got booed all the way off, sat in the dressing room picking at a bit of food, thinking, 'Oh, my fucking Lord!', got booed back on, and then booed back off again five minutes later when we lost. I have never been so embarrassed on a cricket pitch. Thankfully, we didn't see any of the long-suffering England fans outside the ground. In those situations, you just want to keep your head down.

I knew that doubtless we were being slaughtered by the press back in the UK, but it didn't really bother me. Firstly, I was doing OK myself, and secondly, I didn't really care. You know if you play badly you are going to get abused. It didn't bother me because I knew it was going to happen. The travelling fans were different. Unlike the members of the media (and I realise I am now one of them!), they had paid their money and taken their holidays to watch our campaign. Had we not managed to dispatch Scotland in the next game, very possibly there might have been a riot. Against Sri Lanka we found a semblance of form, with me and Joe Root putting together a 98 partnership, but Kumar Sangakkara just brushed us aside. We didn't have the firepower in our bowling attack to compete.

As that World Cup ground to a halt for us, the energy just disappeared from everyone. But I still had hopes of putting in a performance against our penultimate opponents Bangladesh. 'This is going to be great,' I thought. 'This is my time to shine.' I got out for nought and we were careering downhill again. It was always coming. Their tails were up. Ours were dragging on the ground. They bowled us out and that was that. Another World Cup been and gone. I looked on social media after the game – 'Oh my God!' It had all kicked off because Peter Moores had been quoted as saying 'We'll look at the data' following the defeat when in fact he said, 'We'll look at it later'. The media were trying to make out he was some stats-driven robot. Already he'd been painted as someone obsessed with figures and computers and talk. It was unfair. He was much, much more than a numbers drone.

I looked around the dressing room. We were a mess, heads in hands, cringing at the awfulness of the situation. I just wanted to get on the plane – it had been a long winter and we'd been away a long time – but there was one last game, a now meaningless encounter against Afghanistan. My own tournament had gone full circle; the panic measure of putting me at number six hadn't worked and now, with nothing left to play for, I was back batting at three. The game was suitably downbeat, with us getting home via the Duckworth/Lewis method.

We tried to forget our World Cup disaster with a big night out. But there was no escape next morning when, with splitting heads, the management required us to sit round in a circle and give our views on the debacle. No one could escape; everybody was required to say something. Ravi Bopara was the boldest of everybody, which was brave considering he'd been dropped, having barely taken any wickets or scored any runs.

'We're all too weak,' he blasted. 'We're running scared.' He gave it some big licks, proper going hard at everybody. It was fair what he said, but perhaps he wasn't the one to say it!

When it came to my turn to speak, I recognised that ultimately individuals didn't step up. 'We were poor,' I told the room. 'Too often we didn't play as a unit.'

It was a brutal meeting, one of those that the media might term 'clear the air'. Players were going at each other. Coaches were going at players. People were saying exactly what they thought. It was tough – especially with a stinking hangover. But the point was to get things out in the open, to thrash them around. Personally, I don't like problems dealt with that way. It isn't useful. If you've got something constructive to say, fine, but I don't believe in saying things for the sake of it. It's too contrived and can cause resentment. Perhaps we hadn't said enough during the tournament and that's why we were forced to speak. But it was awkward – the most uncomfortable meeting ever.

Moores took a lot of stick during and after the World Cup. He was accused of shackling the team, and that narrative was given some impetus by the more attacking feel to the one day team after he moved on. But that was all so unfair. At that tournament, there were players in the team with scars from previous World Cup failures. Some people doubt this theory, but I'm a definite believer in scars. Having negative preconceived ideas is huge in sport. In a World Cup atmosphere, with games coming quickly one after another, that's not a great place to be.

Personally, I wasn't carrying scars. It could be argued I was only there by accident after Cooky got banned for that game in Sri Lanka. Coming in as I had, and securing my place with 90, backed up with consistently decent scores, meant mentally I was free as a bird. My thinking was nothing more than that – 'I'm doing OK, let's carry it on.' That's how I worked. So often, players complicate matters when they needn't.

Moores gave us freedom if we wanted it – it was more a fact that players in that World Cup team were tainted by past experiences and didn't want to express it. Moores is actually a phenomenal man manager and technician. His energy and passion and love of the game is unbelievable. Wherever he goes he has success in the domestic game. Perhaps his downfall came from not realising that at international level less can be more. Rather than a lot of coaching, players may need help with the mental side of the game, or to have specific sessions set up for them if they need it. At the top level, coaching is a lot more player-led.

At the World Cup, I liked the environment Moores created, but for the senior lads it might not have worked. At the same time, individuals were performing badly, and if individuals aren't performing then the team is going to be rubbish whatever the regime. The team underperforming wasn't Moores' fault, it was the fault of past systems and failures, but he copped the flak for it. Criticism rained down on him from all sides – press and past players.

'He shouldn't be an international coach as he's never played international cricket,' some people claimed. I don't believe that. So long as a coach is helping me, and I trust and respect him, then it's not an issue. I didn't hear any murmurs of that nature from anyone else in that World Cup squad either. Our failing was more about people in the team needing to take a good look at themselves. We needed to sharpen up and pull our finger out, but as a unit we didn't. Truth is, Moores is the most dignified man you will ever meet – another whose career was blighted by Kevin Pietersen, whose arrogance and superiority destroyed him as coach of the England Test team. But you'll never hear Peter Moores say a bad word back. And that says everything for him as a man.

After that World Cup, there had to be change – and there was. New players came in with an open mind. They hadn't been beaten time and again or smashed by the commentators. The likes of Alex Hales and Jason Roy were a totally different breed of attack-minded batsmen with all the latest shots, backed up by a coach saying 'If you want to hit that first ball for six, do it!' Those players had no limiters on them because they hadn't been bashed by the Aussies a dozen times, or smashed by New Zealand on ten occasions. Previous players had negative dour memories. Up until the end of that World Cup I was playing in a one day team where pretty much every time we played, we lost. That creates its own difficulties. It's clearly not going to be a very positive atmosphere. People are constantly going to fear for their places. For this new breed, conversely, it was a case of 'the world's our oyster – let's just go and do it'. Although it wasn't as totally a free rein as some were portraying it, there was a caveat: 'If you mess up the first time, fine. Mess up again, not so good.'

In the current England team, in all formats, not only do they get on well but they also know they're lucky. Sometimes there are players in dressing rooms who have lost an appreciation of what they have. I loved playing for England and everything that came with it – the financial security, the profile, the fans, staying in top-class hotels, having everything done for you. It's a brilliant life. If you want something you can pretty much get it. How many people in everyday life can say that? International sport is amazing, and yet somehow players become jaded, blinkered to the incredibly fortunate life they're leading.

I enjoyed playing for England so much. When the new crop of players got together under the coaching regime of Trevor Bayliss and Paul Farbrace for that first series against New Zealand, I was running on the drinks as twelfth man. With Eoin Morgan away at the Indian Premier League, I'd captained England against Ireland in another rain-affected match in Dublin and hadn't even got to bat, so it seemed a bit tough then to be left out of the side. I should have been angry, have hated carrying those drinks, but actually I was loving it. I loved the atmosphere around the guys and how well they were performing. Just how much fun it was. The change was remarkable. Again, I'm not putting that down to the move from Moores to Farbrace and Bayliss. I'm putting it down to the fact the personnel were so different.

I forced my way back into the team for the one day series against Australia later that summer, and it was at Old Trafford that I realised my ambition of not just an international century, but one against the old enemy. Diving for my ground to reach three figures was something special; especially after getting 98 not out against Australia six months earlier when I should have got a hundred. I loved that Old Trafford knock because it was one that exhibited just what I was all about. I played the situation spot on. As the wickets tumbled at the other end, it was a case of dragging England to a defendable score. Working deliberately and diligently in that cause, I was still scoring at a rate of 90 per 100 balls, but I knew exactly what the commentators would be saying up in their boxes: 'He needs to hurry up here. He's got to crack on.' But they couldn't see what I could – that the pitch was getting worse. I was consciously thinking 'I know what you're saying up there but I'm going to prove you wrong'. And I did – we won by 50 or 60 runs.

I always had that hyper-awareness of what people were saying; I knew what their mindset would be. But I trusted my instinct, my knowledge of the game. The ability to pace a game and an innings can be learned from experience, the difference then is having the balls to carry it through and not panic. OK, you're not going to get it right every time, and in the early days I might have put the team under a bit of pressure by soaking the bowlers up a little too much – hopefully dragging it back later to win the game – but that's fine because as a young player you are gaining knowledge. In time, you learn to tempo an innings, understand the potential of a surface, the size of a ground, who you're up against, what score is achievable. For me, that knowledge came down to playing hundreds of games at all different kinds of levels and knowing exactly what I could deliver. I loved the fact I knew my game so well. Everybody says international cricket is different to county cricket, but if a player knows their game it doesn't have to be. I played my exact same game in international cricket as I did in county cricket. When I got into the England side, it was no different – I could still score in ways that suited my game. I loved my game. I knew it so well. I felt I could get 50 every time I batted, and when I got 50 I felt I could get a hundred. I just stuck to my game plan, went to the options I'd always used, and did it my way.

When Australia batted, the satisfaction when they were losing wickets to our spinners was immense. Having taken some stick off the Aussies in the past, to take them down was really satisfying. David Warner in particular was an average character among average characters. In the first game of the previous winter's tri-series World Cup warm-up tournament against Australia, I got out second ball and he ran up and screamed 'Suck shit, dickhead!' into my face. It didn't end there, but I'd rather not splatter the rest of his expletives across the pages of my book.

Of course, more recently, Warner has been rather more cowed. He's currently serving a year-long ban for his part in the ball-tampering scandal in South Africa. When those pictures first emerged of Cameron Bancroft hiding what turned out to be sandpaper in his trousers, I couldn't believe what I was seeing. This was going way beyond anything I'd witnessed, experienced, or heard of happening on a cricket field. It was obviously a premeditated and calculated attempt to change the condition of the ball by bringing a foreign object on to the field, which is obviously against the rules and spirit of the game.

Don't get me wrong, people do try to change the effect of the ball, or its condition, by doing things on the field. However, it's next level to bring something on to the playing surface to deface the ball, make it move, and try to get an unfair advantage. They had to have thought so far ahead to bring sandpaper on to the field. I could better understand a split second of madness – do what it takes to win – some people can do that and momentarily forget about the consequences. These guys had more than a split second to think about what they were doing, and that's where my sympathy doesn't extend too far.

I did, however, think the sanctions were pretty harsh. A year ban in the context of previous occasions of ball tampering is really extensive. A lot of people have been caught doing it, albeit to a different degree, and they certainly haven't received sanctions half as hard. Already, Steve Smith and Warner have changed their lives forever because they have ruined their reputations, at the same time costing themselves millions. Then to be banned for a year on top of that, as well as losing the captaincy and vice-captaincy of Australia, plus the captaincy of their IPL franchises, is extremely harsh. That's where I do have some sympathy, but at the same time they're both old enough and mature enough to have thought about the consequences.

Even at the original press conference with Smith and Bancroft, it felt like they were too naïve and arrogant to think about the consequences. Yes, they were being honest, but they weren't being 100 per cent honest. It seemed they thought 'If we own up a bit, we'll just get a really big slap on the wrist'. They were too shallow to think about what they'd really done and the context of the game, the spirit of the cricket, and how deep their actions went.

Later, in their individual press conferences, after the full extent of the deceit had come out, Smith and Bancroft showed real emotion. Warner's press conference was interesting to say the least. There was emotion there but he failed to answer a load of questions. I feel for all three from a human point of view. Their lives are over as they know it, and I know what that feels like – although my career was taken away by something out of my control rather than my own stupidity – but in terms of the calculated nature of what they did, then it's a little less easy to feel any pity.

I'm a big believer in doing what it takes to win. However, this was next step. The Australians kept talking about 'headbutting the line'. They were encouraged to be hard on the field, which again is fair, I don't mind that, but they took it to the next level. They did so in the last Ashes. They were incredibly personal to individuals, thinking they could get away with anything. I'm all for doing whatever it takes, but there's a line, and they were teetering on the edge of it consistently. I played against them a lot and they were definitely the toughest opponents. As a cricketer you embrace that challenge; that's exactly how you want it to be. You want your own game to be tested, to be put under pressure, and I would do nothing but compliment their strength as a team. If they did get to me, it was just simple abuse, calling me every name under the sun, abusing me about my height and my ability. OK. That's the way it goes. But to then ratchet it up to include a player's family and personal life? I just don't get it.

There has to be a balance. To me, abuse is pointless. Calling me names – what's the point of that? Getting into the heads of players, dropping little lines in here and there questioning shot selection or technique, is more effective. Paul Nixon at Leicestershire was brilliant at it – a few words and he'd have batsmen second-guessing themselves. That's really powerful – it would have affected me much more than someone abusing me about my height and calling me a twat.

The Aussies, though, seemed to prefer a calculated attack on opponents, something I find really distasteful. When Jonny Bairstow greeted Australia batsman Cameron Bancroft in a bar in Perth in a somewhat unusual manner, a lot was made of the supposed 'headbutt'. They kept on mentioning it in the middle around the stump mic, knowing it would be picked up and a fellow player would get in serious trouble. That needn't have been made public, but the Australians wanted to make something of it. The 'headbutting the line' phrase, coined by Aussie spinner Nathan Lyon, was another dig at Jonny. That sort of thing should be stamped out at the top, but maybe Smith and Lehmann weren't the people to do it. Lehmann appears to like to have enforcers in his teams, while I was always surprised how critical Smith could be towards his players, and the way he spoke to umpires. In that kind of relentlessly harsh environment is it any wonder that lines become blurred as to what is and what isn't acceptable?

Players going at each other is good for the sport. It shows the emotions out there, the passion on display, and the competitive edge. But there's a line. My belief is we'll see a sea change in the Aussies. They won't be as personal or vocal on the field, but they'll still be an incredibly hard team to play. That's great, and that's how they were at Old Trafford that day.

Michael Vaughan called my ton at Old Trafford an 'old school one day century' because I'd worked the ball so well and run the majority of my 101. In the next game at Headingley I showed my versatility, scoring 41 at a run a ball with eight boundaries. I felt invincible, driving the ball on the up, basically playing shots that people never knew I could play, before I was unlucky in getting caught down the leg side. It was a great series for me, one where I'd made real progress, one in which the three lions really began to look good on my chest. I loved playing ODI cricket – such a great way to express your talent and entertain the crowd.

As it was, as I only played twenty-seven ODIs, I never got the chance to reach my peak – that was probably five years away. Even so, alongside my record in other List A cricket matches, I finished fifth in the all-time List A averages behind only Michael Bevan, Virat Kohli, Cheteshwar Pujara and Ab de Fillers – an achievement that still gives me an incredible amount of pride.

As with the rest of my career, when it comes to how far I could have gone in international one day cricket, ultimately I will never know. I'm just thankful for the thrill and the buzz.

Chapter 10

The New Normal

Whenever we were watching TV and a news piece came on about a high profile person having an issue with their heart or dying from a cardiac arrest, it was always the same. I'd turn to Jose: 'I reckon that's going to be me.'

'Oh Jim!' Jose would say. 'Come on!'

Looking back, that's totally bizarre, like there was something inside trying to warn me. I don't believe in that sort of thing, but I do wonder if there was something in my subconscious shouting to be heard – 'I'm so strong, so fit, I've got a perfect life, something has to be wrong.' Even though I was incredibly positive, that tiny little bit of negativity about my own mortality was there.

Mine and Jose's lives are now, rather more consciously, about my mortality. When people say 'It's two years since your attack', they're not entirely correct. It's only as long as it's been since the last scare, the last incident. This is a condition with no magic cure. It's here forever and has a fairly unlikeable habit of reminding me of its presence.

Take last year. I love boxing and was watching the Anthony Joshua versus Wladimir Klitschko world heavyweight fight with some friends. My heart was doing somersaults because I was getting so involved in it, to the extent I had to leave the room. I couldn't be in there anymore. My heart was beating out my chest. All I could do was take my beta-blockers and hope it calmed down. Drugs, as you'd expect, are a constant in my life and always will be. I take pills every morning to slow my heart rate and suppress anxiety. Every time I think I might get nervous or be a little more active then I take more.

If watching other people exert themselves can set me off, then think what my own exercise limits might be. I've never run since that day in April 2016. That's more than two years, and we're talking about someone who exercised all the time. I was in the gym twice a day. I lived for sport. A sportsman was all I ever wanted to be. Now I'm scared of getting the hurry up from a driver while crossing the road. I've been a spectator as the physique I had, that I was so proud of, has slowly disappeared. I was super confident in my body – I was the strongest, the fittest – now that's all gone. Now I'm getting over not having a six-pack, not having the definition on my arms, not having a big chest, my clothes getting baggier. But that's all it is, an ego dent. I'm aware of that. There's nothing I can do about it. I just need to man up and it will be fine. It makes it easier that I don't want to go to the gym. It's not like I'm being stopped, or don't have time – I physically can't. That's easier to get my head around.

I'd like to say I compensate for the lack of exercise by eating differently. Truth is, I eat utter rubbish. I'm chewing my way through a Galaxy bar right now. Occasionally I used to cook when I lived on my own, but a lot of the time I'd eat out seven days a week – breakfast, lunch and dinner. Now I'm a bit more aware financially! And eating out all the time isn't good for you anyway – for your wallet or your wealth. Jose is aware of my weakness for junk and so tries to make me have my five a day every day. She'll cook something healthy and then hand me some fruit.

Thankfully, my metabolism is good from being a sportsman. When I came out of hospital, Jose encouraged me to keep eating to maintain that metabolism. It was clearly going to slow down, but the idea was, while it was working, keep it working. I'm doing really well to stay thin but I'm paranoid about putting on weight. I always have been – another factor that drove me to get fitter and stronger and look better. I always put myself down so I'd work harder. It was like batting – I always told myself I looked worse than I actually did to make myself work harder. It all stems from fear of failure. My entire cricket career was based on a fear of failure.

My heart has not ever let me forget its presence. When the soreness from the defib operation had calmed down, I still had an odd sensation. It felt like I was being continually flicked on the inside of my chest, a tiny little tap, persistent. The defib was supposed to be another step towards being able to live without the constant nagging, gnawing awareness of my condition, and yet here I was with a mentally very unsettling reminder. No escape. When it became clear it wasn't going to go away, we saw John Walsh. He got it straight away.

'Well, that's a constant reminder of everything,' he pondered. 'You can't live like that.'

Thankfully, the defib can be controlled externally – I wouldn't be going back under the knife. John worked out a way to stop the flicking without compromising the device. Such a brilliant doctor. But it still happens roughly once a week – a reminder that there is something there inside my body. A reminder I'd rather not have.

Social interruptions aren't unusual. At a wedding we were having a great time, enjoying the company of friends, laughing and joking. Suddenly I turned to Jose. 'My heart's not right.' We had to leave, assess where I was at. And there you are, straight back down to earth.

The most innocuous things can set me off. Recently I was watching a war film. Jose could see the pulse in my neck going. 'Jim, just pause it if you need to!'

Everything I drink I have to think twice about. Caffeine, obviously, is a no-no (shame because I always liked a Coke!), but food has to be on my radar too. I had a firecracker chicken from Wagamama and that set me off. Spices, you see – I have to take care. No wonder sometimes I just like to sit down with something non-threatening like a bar of Galaxy.

Occasionally, Jose and I just forget where we're at. We always used to make each other jump, leaping out of doorways or waiting at the top of the stairs. Jose did it not long after we came out of hospital – it was so automatic. As soon as she did it, she couldn't believe it – 'What am I doing?'

But I'm no better. I still run up the stairs. It's how I'm programmed. I stopped for a while – at first every time I went upstairs I'd panic – but old habits die hard and now I never ever walk up the stairs. When I get to the top I wait for a second. Am I all right? Oh, OK. Carry on.

Cars are a danger area. Think how often you have little, or maybe major, irritations while you're out on the road. I was with Jose, who, thankfully, is really careful, when another driver objected to her pulling out in front of him and accelerated to an inch from her bumper with his lights on full beam and horn blaring. That's not great at any time, even more so when you've got someone in the car who could potentially have a heart attack. I can't get angry, I just can't.

Another time, someone stopped dead right in front of her. She slammed the break on and the belt jerked and pulled so tight against me, right where my defib is positioned. A horrible feeling. Again, scary.

The worst for me is noises. Gunshots on TV, bangs, anything like that. 'Was that my defib?' It takes me a whole five seconds of silence to ascertain exactly what has happened. That might sound daft, but imagine if you had something in your chest that goes 'Bang!' when it goes off. I assure you that you'd be just the same.

Friends are great. I don't want them tiptoeing around me, treading on eggshells, and generally we just get on with everything as normal. Occasionally, though, they'll forget. A mate recently suggested we go skiing.

'I can't, it's an activity.'

People are horrified when something like that happens, and I never want anyone to feel bad. It's exactly the kind of thing I'd do if the boot was on the other foot! They're still training their brains to be ARVC-sensitive just the same as I'm training mine. Even now, I'll stand up too quickly, which makes me feel really dizzy, as if I'm going to faint. It happens pretty much once a day. Low blood pressure as a result of my beta-blockers causes that situation.

One situation, though, was on a different level from a little light-headedness when rising from a table. In fact, it was the scariest incident in the whole time since my heart condition came to light – including the day it all kicked off in Cambridge.

It was a year on from that day when Steve Schofield asked me if I'd accompany him as a coach on a tour to Antigua with a team from Maidwell Hall. It made for a neat circle. It was exactly the same tour as the first one I'd ever been on as a 13-year-old. Now here I was coaching alongside the very same man who took me over there – same resort, same hotel, same pitches, everything. After a tough year, it appealed to me in lots of ways. Head over to the Caribbean, do some coaching, feel the sun on my back, and all in a place I'd loved as a kid.

Initially, it was everything I thought it would be. Steve was great company, there was plenty of time to relax, and at the same time I was investing in a future in coaching. We'd get the boys up early and take them running on the beach, then we'd have breakfast, a net, and go and chill in the hotel pool.

We were chatting away in the water, leaning on the edge of the pool.

'How many hundreds did you get in your career?'

'Shedloads.'

'OK, how many?'

'Eighty-five.'

I knew my hundreds right back to when I was eleven. I used that statistic as a reminder of how much effort I'd put in.

'And that's without all the 80s and 90s!'

At that moment, from nowhere, I was propelled at rocket speed 10 feet back through the water. I was dazed, confused. I couldn't understand what had happened. Steve was as shocked as I was. He thought maybe I'd been stung by an insect.

It took me a few seconds to realise that my defib had gone off. I couldn't believe it. If my defib had gone off when all I'd been doing was relaxing in a pool, then my heart really must be messed up. I was hoping it was an inappropriate shock, that the defib had reacted with something in the vicinity. Or perhaps the position of my left arm as I held on to the poolside had caused it to behave unusually.

Steve helped me out of the pool and we walked back to my room, pondering the consequences. How bad was it? Would I have to go home? Would I lose my driving licence again? I wasted no time. I had a little computer that downloaded information from my defib. Straight away I sent it to the hospital in Nottingham. Ten minutes later, I followed it up with a phone call. The medics confirmed it was an inappropriate shock. My defib wasn't meant to go off. It must have reacted with something in the pool. I thought back and remembered where I was leaning was a gobbler, a filter that pumps water out of the pool. I'd been told from the start to stay away from equipment such as generators because they can cause havoc with the rhythm of a defib, and a pump is similar in many ways. Steve later took pictures of the hotel's two pools for the doctors to see. The colour of one was different from the other. Perhaps a pump in one pool was faulty or inefficient; either way it had definitely affected me.

The hospital said I could stay in Antigua if I wanted. It made sense. I only had three more days, and my defib had gone off by accident anyway. It hadn't gone off because of an issue with my heart. I went down from my room and did some gentle coaching. Bearing in mind my heart had just had several hundred volts put through it, and had just been restarted, I wasn't going to do anything too strenuous. I made sure to take a long diversion around the guilty swimming pool.

That evening, Steve and I went for a swim in the sea. I felt a little bit shaken by what had happened earlier, but it wasn't weighing on my mind. I was in a clear blue sea in Antigua chatting with an old pal – what's not to like?

We headed back to the hotel, happy in the knowledge that it would be same again tomorrow, and as I lay on my bed sleep came naturally.

At 3.00 am I woke with a start. There was an alarm going off. Blearily, I got up, searching everywhere for what was making the noise. I was looking under the bed, in drawers, in the bathroom, behind the wardrobe. I was totally baffled. 'Where is it coming from?'

Thirty seconds later, I realised.

'Fuck! It's my defib.'

A sick feeling was rising in my throat. To have this machine wailing away inside me was awful.

'Oh God, no! It's broken.'

By now my heart was bursting from my chest. I couldn't believe it. Horrifically, it was right back in the rhythm that I'd suffered a year previously when I thought I was going to die. I was back on the same nightmarish ride, consumed by that same absolute fear, the all-encompassing despair of impending death.

I sat on the floor of the bathroom praying, pleading for my defib to spring into life. When that didn't work I lay in the floor instead. Bizarre to think I'd spent all my time since it was fitted hoping more than anything that my defib wouldn't fire into life and now here I was desperate for it to blast me across the room. Basically, I was lying on a bathroom floor in Antigua waiting for my chest to explode.

Previously, when the defib had gone off at Leicester, it had all happened too quickly for me to register. This time was different – I was reliving the horror of that original day. It was the same beat, the same feeling, the horror of my heart trying to smash through my chest. I was doing it all again – only this time with nobody to save me.

At least the first time it happened I was in England. There were people equipped to help me – even it did take me a while to get to them. Now here I was, at 3.00 am, in Antigua, with a broken defib, seemingly having a heart attack, and there was nobody. The hospital was miles away and wouldn't have the same facilities as Nottingham anyway. All I could think was 'I'm screwed'.

'My pills.' I fetched my wash bag, got them out, and essentially overdosed, because what was going on in my chest was so extreme, I thought it was the only possible way to calm my heart down. It didn't. My heart was still going mad, but I did compose myself enough to download the defib readings to the hospital back in Nottingham.

I Facetimed Jose. My eyes were wide. 'My heart's racing,' I said. 'It's happening all over again. My defib's alarming. It's making an ambulance sound. I'm scared. I want it to shock. It's not working.' I could feel my heart rate going up and up.

I didn't tell her, but I'd rung to say goodbye. I didn't want to panic her, but at the same I was consciously thinking what I wanted the last thing I'd say to her to be.

'Just know I love you,' I told her as the tears came. 'Just know I love you.' She knew what I was doing, knew what I was trying to say, and wasn't going to acknowledge it. To acknowledge it would have made it even more real.

'It will be all right,' she kept telling me. 'Everything is going to be OK.'

But all I could think was that if my defib was broken and I was having a heart attack in Antigua in the middle of the night, I was going to die. In this scenario, what was going to save me?

My heart felt like it was going a million miles an hour, thumping into the side of my chest. Over and over again I told her I loved her. I wanted her to know what she meant to me, and always had. More than anything, I wanted her to be with me. I wanted to close those 5,000 miles and have her by my side. She was the one who could get me back down to where I needed to be. She was the one who could help me survive.

Back in the UK, because of the time difference, Jose was stood in a classroom with a load of Year 11 teenagers outside the door trying to get in. On the other end of the phone she had her husband saying goodbye because he thought he was about to die. 'Get Steve in your room,' she told me.

I woke Steve up to come and sit with me. I knew I needed to calm down. 'Steve's here,' I told her.

That meant, against all her instincts, she could hang up and call the hospital. In tears, she ran down from the classroom through the hustle and bustle of those early morning corridors to get someone to cover her class. The staffroom emptied as she frantically tried to get through to the hospital. Thankfully, there was someone on duty. They said they'd have a look at the readings and call her back.

Still nothing from my defib. In my head it was broken. Minutes passed. Nothing. All the time Steve was trying to comfort me, to talk about anything to take my mind, even for a second, away from what was happening in my chest.

Within minutes, the hospital rang Jose back. 'We're tracing his heart rate now,' a doctor told her. There was a pause. 'It's fine. It's in rhythm.'

She rang me straight away. Never have I been gladder to hear two words – 'in rhythm'. That was the key – it didn't matter if my heart was going fast so long as it was in rhythm. Jose was so excited to tell me.

'Are you sure?' I asked. 'Are you sure? Is that what they said? Do you promise?' I was clinging on to her words.

'Yes, I promise. It's fine.' The relief was overwhelming.

The reason my defib was alarming, the doctor said, was because I'd been shocked but then hadn't had it reset at hospital. As a reminder, it went off after fifteen hours. The problem was I wasn't aware of this routine. I didn't even know the defib had a siren. And so there I was, at 3.00 am, in a hotel room in Antigua, having a meltdown, thinking I was having a heart attack, that I was going to die – and all for no apparent reason. Slowly my heart was getting back to normal as the pills kicked in, although even thirty-five to forty minutes later it was still playing tricks with me. Steve stayed with me as I returned to something resembling my usual self. He told me he was thinking he might have to perform CPR, and that Jose's strength was incredible.

He was right. Jose, yet again, had been my lifesaver. She knew before she'd even picked the phone up that it was going to be serious. I knew she'd be at school, so why else would I ring at that time? I was lucky she answered. Five minutes later and she'd have put her phone away in a drawer so as not to distract her from teaching.

We acknowledged afterwards the true nature of that call.

'Did you know how close to dying I thought I was?' I asked.

'Yes, yes, I did. I knew you were saying goodbye.'

That's me and Jose. Anyone else listening to that conversation would never have known.

Once I'd calmed down, there was only one thing that mattered to me – getting home. If my defib was going to alarm every fifteen hours, I couldn't be in Antigua, around people, when the next one happened. How embarrassing would that be? We're not talking a little phone alarm here. This thing would quite adequately clear a building in a fire. Imagine that coming from inside you. More importantly, if it did alarm again there was every chance it would set my heart off on another episode of craziness, like it had during the night.

I tried to get a flight to the UK. There weren't any. Eventually, however, I found one that was premium economy. It was extortionate – £1,600 for a one-way flight. Steve told one of the parents of the young Maidwell tourists and he spread the word, and before I knew it a group of mums and dads had clubbed together to get me home. Truly incredible kindness.

A whole day had passed by the time I reached the airport. It was crunch time for the defib. I was sat in departures just waiting for it to alarm. That wait then continued on the plane. I was in my seat expecting it to go off at any time. I felt it wise to explain in advance to the person in the next seat. But then how exactly do you tell someone, 'Excuse me, but any time now you might hear an alarm go off. Don't worry, it's just me. It's in my chest.'

In the end, I got chatting with the woman just to make small talk, so I would eventually be in a position to break the news. Thankfully, there was no need. It never went off. Mum picked me up straight from the airport and we headed to the hospital to have it reset.

I haven't been in a pool since. Actually, that's a lie. In Adelaide last winter, it was so hot outside the hotel that I just leapt into the pool. Crazy really, because I'd already made sure not to sit too near the pumps or filters. I jumped in, thought about it, and then jumped straight out again. It didn't make any sense to take the risk.

I've been specifically told to stay away from bubble pools, and in fact if I'm near anything with a pump I'm seriously worried. At a petrol station, I'm stood as far away as I can from the pump, filling my car with my arm stretched out. People must think I'm mad, but the way I see it, if my defib has gone off once because of a pump, what's to stop it happening again?

After Antigua, petrol pumps weren't an issue. I lost my licence again due to a defib ruling by the DVLA. After the first attack I lost it for six months. Three months into that, I had the incident at the Q&A, which meant the six months started again from scratch. This time, thankfully, it was only for a month because it was an external influence that had set it off.

If I didn't lose my licence, I'd maybe push myself more physically. But having lost so much, I really don't want to lose my independence as well. Six months without driving is tough. It's just not worth it.

That trepidation, that constant re-educating, will be with us forever. Commentating on England games in Australia and New Zealand last winter, I always had to be on my guard when entering stadia. Just like at Twickenham, I can't have them wave that detector wand over me because it will affect my defib. If I don't spot that guard before they spot me then it's too late. It's the same when I fly – I can't go through the scanners. The staff are clued up for people like me; I point at my chest and they know straight away.

So much of my new life is about knowing my limits. I was in Australasia for two months. You can't do that kind of trip with hand luggage. My bag was so heavy and there was always a nagging thought at the back of my mind that lugging it from flight to flight, hotel to hotel, might not be a great idea. Same with coaching – I have to rein myself in massively. It doesn't hamper what I do, but it does stop me doing it to the nth degree. Without ARVC I would certainly be a lot more dynamic, but I don't gamble anymore. For me it would be like a game of Russian roulette. I've never been a gambler in the past and I certainly don't intend starting now.

Slowly, Jose and I are rebuilding our confidence when it comes to living our lives. When we first came out of hospital, we stepped back and thought about every single thing. Now we're more assured. Even so, I'll never have an hour when I don't think about my heart. Every time I go up the stairs, every time I do any activity, every time I get up, I think about it. Even bed offers no escape. I can't start off lying on my left because I can feel the defib – and that makes me think about my heart. From nowhere I've got a mental and physical discomfort. Even sleep itself offers no escape. I have nightmares about my defib going off. I wake up with a start and it takes me a good thirty seconds to realise it's a dream. My heart, though, will be going nuts because of the adrenalin of the nightmare. Off I go to the bathroom and take my beta-blockers.

Alcohol, or rather the lack of it, has been another big change. Obviously, I'm in my twenties. Pre-ARVC I enjoyed a drink. Now I barely touch it. I can have a drink but I rarely do because it increases my heart rate. That feeling of waking up in the middle of the night, my heart thumping away, like a sledgehammer smacking into my ribs, just isn't worth it. I don't want to take a self-inflicted bullet.

Not drinking anymore, the hardest thing in those first six months was finding a release. Alcohol was a no-no – and that had always been my number one escape, going out on a bender and forgetting about life's pressures. The way I saw it, though, not being able to drink was a blessing in disguise. At such a traumatic time, it would have been all too easy to have hit the bottle, which would then have meant losing control of what I needed to do to maintain my health and could also have affected my relationship with Jose.

The gym had always been another release – I couldn't do that. Sport was a release – I couldn't do that. What can I do? Finding that one release was really tough. The one thing I could do was watch live sport, which I loved. I'd go to the races, tennis, football, rugby. But there was still the element of participation missing. Another option, though, was rapidly forming in my mind – golf.

It had always been a sport I wanted to take up and after the defib was fitted I went about pursuing it seriously. Sadly, I was hindered initially by not being able to swing a club because my defib hadn't yet set properly behind my muscle. I would feel it getting squeezed and moving when I tried to swing. By October, though, it had set, and that was the first time I could play golf. It changed my life. A new challenge, a new technique to learn, something competitive that I could throw myself at. I'd only ever played a little bit up until I was twelve, so I was basically taking it from scratch. On the driving range I was great. Then I'd get on the course and I'd be awful. I was so embarrassed. But I ploughed on, challenging myself, driving myself on – 'You've got to get better!'

Golf now is an absolute passion, bordering, Jose would say, on an obsession. I'd be on a course every waking moment if it were possible. It's been a huge saviour; a living connection with a love of sport that I thought from now on would be unrequited. Where do you go when your job, your whole raison d'être, is as a sportsman, and then it's taken away? 'Sportsman' is a word that defines everything about you. A word that portrays attitude and aptitude, a pursuit of brilliance. A word that encompasses everything I am. Not was – am. I lost many things on 6 April 2016, but a love of sport and a desire to participate was not one of them. I'm not saying I'm going to be the next Open champion, but golf has put some tangible purpose back into my sporting life.

The target is to get to scratch and play in the biggest tournaments I can, just to get a little bit of something – the limelight, the sporting environment, whatever you want to call it. That's what I miss – being that person who people come to watch. I've always had that side of me that enjoys showing off. I miss that a lot. I miss people coming up to me wanting my autograph – that selfish, ego side of sport. I miss being the best in the room. When that gets taken away, it's a big ego dent.

Golf has made me feel like me again. And that's what I want more than anything. I can make my way in this new world just fine, but I'd enjoy it even more if I was accompanied by some elements of my former self. The old me never died. He just needs to know how he fits into the new me.

My life has changed and it hasn't changed. I'm different but I'm not different. It can start to give you a headache if you think about it too much.

I have an easier way to describe it – the new normal.

Chapter 11

Short Leg

They say that all good things come to those who wait, although I was beginning to wonder at the wisdom of that saying when it came to my Test career. Eventually, though, my chance to re-establish myself as a Test player did come.

The century against Australia, in which I'd shown the versatility of my technique, hitting just five 4s in accruing 101, had clearly counted in my favour. I'd also had a golden end to the summer, scoring 555 runs in my last five Championship matches. With my reputation as a good player of spin, a tour to the UAE against Pakistan was right up my street, and finally the selectors agreed. Now, it seemed, was my time. Even so, it took Jos Buttler to hit a poor run of form to create a space for me in the team for the third Test. I used the time in between to speak to Alastair Cook, who would obviously have had a big influence in selection as captain, about my years in the wilderness. When I was twelfth man for the second Test, I had a playful conversation with the skipper. I was taking the Mick, saying I should have played more. To be fair, Cook openly admitted that he'd hardly seen me play in the longer format. I'd scored a hundred against Essex when I was nineteen, and 62 in the second innings, when he was playing, but that was about it. Andy Flower, the England coach for much of the time when I was out in the cold, was the same. The combination of the two not seeing me enough was probably detrimental. They had no real idea of the capacity to which I could play, and that was automatically going to go against me.

While it wasn't ideal that I played so many games for the Lions, the positive side was that when I did eventually come back into the full England team I was totally ready and prepared. I'd played against so many full international sides and scored runs against them I knew for sure I could play at that level. That, allied to my desperation to score runs, was a good combination. I'd been waiting so long to get back into Test cricket, it felt like my debut again – the same excitement, the same desire to perform. Except now I was more confident because I'd done well in the ODIs and cemented myself in that side.

As I walked out to bat at Sharjah, I had one big thought in my mind when it came to those who hadn't picked me for all those years: 'I want to show you what you've been missing.' And that's exactly what I did. I made 74 on a ragged pitch in the toughest of tough conditions – heat, humidity, and high quality spin bowling. The ball was turning square, but it suited me. Fast feet meant I could get either close to the ball or far away, and my low centre of gravity meant I was agile and could react quickly. I never feared playing spin; I loved the challenge, and that made the difference. Other people would get stuck and then get out. I also loved the fact that for a lot of that innings I had Jonny at the other end. We batted well together and injected a new lease of life into the team. We knew each other, the way we ran between the wickets, the intensity with which we both played.

In all honesty, I should have played every Test that tour. I'd scored runs in the warm-up and the selectors knew I could play spin, whereas a lot of the lads weren't the best. I perhaps should also have opened. They would never have contemplated opening with me in England, but in Dubai, where the Kookaburra ball doesn't do much and there was going to be a lot of spin, it would have been a good option. They went with Moeen Ali in the end, which was frustrating, but understandable as Mo was already opening in the one day team.

Either way, my performance in Sharjah bought me a ticket on the plane for the second half of the winter in South Africa. It felt, at last, like I was a proper England Test player. When you become established, you get a different reaction from those around you; there's more respect for what you can do, and that's how I now felt. Ever since I came back into the full England setup, I'd been contributing. Succeeding in international cricket, proving wrong the people who didn't think I could do it, was just an amazing feeling. It gave me confidence to express myself even more.

Not only that, but we felt tight as a group. Many of us had come through together and were sharing new experiences, wanting to succeed, and playing off each other's successes. It felt like we all wanted the same thing, and supported each other, rather than egos getting in the way – talking of which, KP had been dropped for good following the Ashes drubbing of 2013/14. Of course, there were still egos around, but not to the detriment of the side. These were players thinking 'I'm going to show off' rather than 'I'm going to belittle somebody'. It's arrogance in the right way. Swagger rather than hammer. Positive arrogance is the embodiment of confidence; it's necessary sometimes to be able to impose yourself on the game and also the opposition. When I was really grafting and determined, or was taking the bowling on, then I had a little bit of arrogance. But you would never see Alastair Cook playing with arrogance. He didn't need to. He had a natural superiority of talent.

It was the same with getting hit. I didn't get hit much but when I did it gave me something extra. It would give me a shake and take me to another level. If anything, it would make me more dogged. Some people might shy away after being hurt, but for me it got me concentrating. It brought out an extra layer of spirit. Arrogance, so long as it doesn't tip over into complacency, can do exactly the same.

Arrogance on its own, though, will get a player nowhere. It is the snow-topped peak on a mountain of knowledge. I always knew where I needed to score against every single bowler before I went in. For the first Test match against South Africa in Durban, I walked into bat and the right arm spinner Dane Piedt was on. Piedt was relatively new to Test cricket but I had studied him, so I wasn't as nervous as I might otherwise have been. I knew my game plan and what I needed to do. When I saw the South Africans had placed long-on out towards the boundary for my first ball, to me that was brilliant. I knew I could just trot down and knock Piedt out to that fielder for an easy single and there I was, off the mark in the series, job done. I had clarity of vision, which made a massive difference. Clarity delivers absolute certainty. When you're questioning yourself and not as confident, that's when your game breaks down, especially if you haven't the perfect technique. I didn't have the perfect technique but I could deal with most challenges well enough. My mind, awareness and cricketing knowledge could cover any flaw in my technique. Questioning yourself out in the middle reduces your performance to 60 per cent of what it should be. I never saw the point of clouding my focus. I never liked to hear batsmen in the dressing room talking about specific bowlers – 'He's turning it square', 'How quick is he bowling?' That's a negative thought process. It's almost like you're finding readymade excuses for when it goes wrong. My view was, 'The more skilful the bowler, the better I'm going to look when I take him down', not 'How bad am I going to look if I mess up?' I always wanted to play against the best. I never felt intimidated by or scared by a bowler – I loved the challenge. I faced Mitchell Johnson when he was bowling at 90mph-plus and I would have loved to have faced Brett Lee or Shoaib Akhtar just to see what it was like. People say nobody likes short-pitched bowling, but I did as it was an opportunity for me to score. I used to relish taking it on because it was a strength of mine. And taking on a fight is a way of deflecting the pressure in your head. Irritatingly, while I had the measure of the pace and spin merchants, it was the slow metronomic bowlers, the guys who could move it around, who caused me trouble and tested my technique. Give me the Rawalpindi Express any day of the week.

That single down to long-on turned into a vital knock of 70 at a time when we were under pressure against one of the best sides in the world. I added another 42 in the second innings as we beat the South Africans by 241 runs. It was an amazing feeling to know I'd fronted up and made a difference, and confirmed again, after my 76 in the previous Test in Pakistan, that I was good enough to play at the very highest level.

The way to cement your position in any side is to do as much as you can to make yourself indispensable. My athleticism in the field had always worked in my favour from that point of view, and when it came to England I wanted to add as many strings as I could to my bow. In South Africa this personified itself in my taking a key position at short leg and making it absolutely my own. I was totally proactive in that move and worked tirelessly with Paul Farbrace to get as good at it as I could. I was still suffering shoulder pain and so wasn't able to perform as I'd have liked in the outfield. My thought process was simple: 'I'm going to be in the ring anyway, so I might as will get good at it.' And it suited me. I loved being in the thick of the action and would always much rather be close in than out in the deep being bored somewhere.

I'd always worked hard at my close-in fielding skills but now I began really nailing them, and it soon paid off. In the first innings of the third Test at Johannesburg I was caught by Temba Bavuma, a really good catch above his head off Morné Morkel. My immediate thought was, 'Forget you, I'm going to do something really special. I'm going to get people looking at me.' And that's exactly what happened. In South Africa's second innings, I was so focused I genuinely believed I could catch anything. I did things I'd never done before that day. Hashim Amla was the first, and I still think of all the close catches I took in that series – it was the best. It was a proper shot, a well-timed flick off the legs that should in reality have been past me before I even saw it. The time the ball took from his bat to my hands was timed later at 0.4 of a second. Catching a rocket doesn't just happen. To track the batsman's movements, and to time your own movements correctly, is a skill in itself. You can't just stand there. You need trigger movements, just as you do as a batsman. You have to follow the ball from the bowler's arm, look at the batsman's body position, identify where the ball is potentially going to go, and then think, 'Right, what position do I need to be in if I'm going to catch this?' There are a million things going on, but you just do it naturally because, if you've practised correctly, you've trained your body to react in the right way.

With Amla, that split second of catching the ball and then waiting for everyone to cheer – confirmation that it really had happened – was unbelievable. It almost felt like my wicket, because it wouldn't have happened without me. I set off on this amazing run. And it wasn't just me; everybody else was going mad too. Ben Stokes high-fived me mid-air as we both ran at each other. I saw a photograph later and he's going so fast his feet don't touch the ground for several metres. He might have thought about a career as a long jumper.

That feeling was the best I've ever had on a cricket field. It reminds me of my wedding. It's not every day you look round and see everybody smiling, but that was one of those times. The camaraderie, the celebration, it was brilliant. I'm so glad I did that before I finished.

To then do it again six overs later, this time diving to my right and almost behind me to pluck the ball out of the air and see off Dane Vilas, was unbelievable. It showed everyone that the first catch wasn't a fluke – that this was something I had specifically worked at to become an expert – especially when in the next game at Centurion I took another great short leg catch, this time catching Dean Elgar between my legs, having again tracked the batsman's movement to ensure I was in the absolute perfect position to take the chance.

Short leg is a position of the finest of fine margins. You've got less than half a second to make the decision whether to stay upright, because it might pop up, or tuck up in a ball because it's coming straight at you right off the middle. The instinct that helps you catch the ball is the same one that gets you into a safe position – head covered, arms and hands tucked in. If you're scared then it's not something you're going to be able to do. I was lucky in that I hadn't been hit a lot in my career fielding in that position, and because I was generally the youngest and smallest in most teams I played in, I'd been shoved there a lot. Yes, I'd been hit, but never anything that had caused me too much trouble. I'd never broken any bones, let's put it like that.

It's rare that a player works so hard on one element of the game and it pays off straight away, but it just shows the benefits of never sitting still and accepting your lot. As a batsman there will be games where you don't score many, and then you've got to bring something extra to the team. It always really annoyed me when I saw players offering nothing. Fielding is something I've always enjoyed, but my view was I could give more to it. I looked at it not just from my point of view, but the batsman's. I knew from my own experience that when there are really good fielders around, it adds a little something extra to a batsman's mental load.

What I did in South Africa reaffirmed what a vital position short leg is. You need to take twenty wickets to win a Test match. If you've got a player who can, quite literally, pluck a couple from thin air, then they soon become worth their weight in gold – which in my case isn't very much, but you see what I mean!

I loved playing in that team. After all those years of trying to make a breakthrough, I was there at last, alongside my peers who'd travelled the same road but without the hold-ups. Root was a great example, a good lad who is a really great player, not brash or outlandish but grounded and level-headed – similar to me in many ways. Root is a player who leads by example. But when he was given the captaincy I worried for him because of the big personalities in that England side. Cooky wouldn't be a problem – it's not in his nature – but that still left the likes of Jimmy and Broady, great characters and fantastic players, but maybe slightly intimidating for a young captain seeking to make his mark. In his favour, Root had always spoken up in team meetings, and that background would make it easier. And being a batsman, of course, he wouldn't pose a threat.

With Jonny, meanwhile, I saw a guy who could play the shots and hit the ball incredibly hard, and another who had needed to prove to others that he could perform consistently at the top level. Did he have the discipline or the technique to back it up? He certainly had the mental toughness. From a boy, when he lost his dad, the former England wicketkeeper David Bairstow, he'd shown an incredible strength. If I wanted somebody to bat for my life, Jonny might not be technically perfect, but I know he'd always step up to the occasion.

It was crazy the amount of fuss that was made over the head butt incident on the last Ashes tour of Australia when Jonny greeted Australia batsman Cameron Bancroft in a bar in Perth in a somewhat unusual manner. It was just Jonny being Jonny. The fact it was called a head butt made it sound much worse than it actually was. It was just a light-hearted, if a bit clumsy, touching of heads. Thing is, when a team is losing, incidents like that become a big deal. When a team is winning, the media is more willing to laugh them off.

Pinning any kind of blame for England's 4–1 Ashes loss in Australia on a drinking culture was crazy.

Australia had got players in form – all their pacemen plus their spinners. England had Dawid Malan and Jonny Bairstow in form and Jimmy bowling nicely. That's three out of eleven. If people weren't blaming booze, it was county cricket's fault. Really? It was nothing to do with county cricket, it was about individuals being in form and being ready, and a host country, just as we do, exploiting its own conditions.

After the Stokes episode in Bristol there's now a magnifying glass on every single player. I was captain of the Lions when Stokes got sent home from Australia – he loved the country too much and just wanted constantly to be out and having fun. I didn't mind him and his mate, the Kent paceman Matt Coles, going out drinking so long as they performed. Stokes would drink when he shouldn't be drinking, but when he turned up at the ground the next day there was nobody who would train more intensely. Some players would slack off but that never happened with Stokes. What annoys me is when others who have had too many drinks cruise by the wayside. You've got to throw everything you can into your playing, because there's nothing quite like being a professional sportsman. Away from the pitch, as long as it's not going to impact on your playing and training, enjoy yourself as much as you can. On that Lions tour, Stokes went out once too often. He pushed his luck and it backfired on him when Andy Flower felt he needed teaching a lesson. I had no input into the decision to send him home. With the Lions, I was captain but it wasn't my team. It's not like being the full England captain where your influence invades all areas.

What's often needed is a mentor, and that's why I always went back to those people who'd looked after me, shaped me, and pushed me in the right direction. The bollocking I had off Paul Pridgeon at Shrewsbury always lived with me because I never wanted to let people down. My career was for other people as well as me. Don't get me wrong, as an England player I'd drink, but I did it under the radar. I never wanted to be in a situation where it could affect my selection. I made sure my preparation as a cricketer was never affected. I always practised hard. When I was with England I was better than most. I trained my tits off, as they say. I used Cook as a target, because he was super fit. We did our annual fitness tests together, and the last time out I beat him – success after so many years.

There's always a balance. Sometimes you get it wrong, other times you get it right. In my eyes, you should do whatever you can to become a better player, but at the same time never forget to have fun. I sacrificed a lot, missed out on so many parties in my teenage years because I was playing the next day, but I also had my fair share of blow-outs. I found the balance. Nowadays it's tough for youngsters. When I travelled with the U-19s to the World Cup in Malaysia, we went out a lot, but when I coached the U-19s in South Africa last year, it was like being back at school. They couldn't do anything. It was that strict. I was on duty some nights as they had to sign in and sign out and I couldn't help thinking of my own antics at Shrewsbury once or twice. We had to look after them – can you imagine if anything had happened with the U-19s on top of everything that had happened with the England team?

International players have to recognise that they live in a world of instant recognition, of mobile phones, of people who may see their presence as a challenge. When incidents do happen I always hear people ask why there wasn't protection, security officers accompanying players on nights out. Usually there are, but it's no solution. Players will sneak off and do their own thing. They're grown men – it's nobody else's fault but their own. There's only so much that security guards can do when faced with young lads who are drunk and want to get away from them.

There are other ways of enjoying the camaraderie of top-level sport. After the final Test at Centurion, the two teams had a fines meeting. We all had to fine each other and Morné Morkel was the fines master. I was fined for not being the smallest – Bavuma was even smaller than me. It was brilliant fun as all the players and coaching staff had a drink together. AB de Villiers and a couple of other South African players stayed in the England dressing room before some of the Barmy Army came in and we all sung songs to the accompaniment of the trumpeter – even AB was joining in.

That South Africa trip was my big breakthrough moment. I'd been given the opportunity I so longed for and I'd taken it. I felt like finally I'd gone beyond the seemingly endless rigmarole of wondering if I'd be picked or again left out in the wilderness. We won the series when we weren't expected to, and I contributed. I felt very happy and comfortable in myself as an England cricketer, and my game was in such a good place that it was only natural that I felt I'd be there when it came to the first Test of the season against Sri Lanka. That particular opportunity, of course, was denied to me. But South Africa was such a good way to go out – having the time of my life, playing Test cricket, and winning a Test series, while surrounded by some great lads, on both sides.

Looking back on my England career, I see it as almost the embodiment of myself. You could say the stars never quite aligned for James Taylor and international cricket – six of my seven Test matches were against South Africa, the number one team in the world, and my first eighteen one day internationals were away. But when the clouds blocked out a perfect constellation, I was always a big believer in finding a way to blow them clear. That's no different in life. England might have gone but when I look at the night sky now, those stars are crystal clear.

Chapter 12

Jose

When we got into the back of my mum's car on 6 April 2016, Jose immediately clutched my hand. It was an early indication of what was to come, the strength and love within her. She's held me close ever since.

I didn't know Jose at all at school. I knew all the girls in her year but she never went out. She always had her head in a book, studying, improving, super intelligent. I'd left school by the time I met her. It was November, her birthday, when we first spoke in a club. I was eighteen, she was seventeen. I had no idea what an integral part of my life she would become. I had met the person who made me complete.

It's difficult to comprehend what my life would have been like without Jose before the incident in Cambridge. It's even harder to comprehend now. If I didn't have Jose, I genuinely don't know what I'd do, where I'd be. We've always been unbelievably close – anyone will tell you that – but since that day when everything changed we've been on a different level. We know each other inside out. She senses even the slightest issue with my heart. Body movements, expressions – when I feel anything happen inside of me, she knows. Bearing in mind what happened to me was originally thought to be a virus, she should never really have come home that day when it all started. But she knew it was something more serious, because she knows me better than even I know myself.

Any concerns at all, however minor they might appear, she wants me to tell her. That way we can work through them together. I'll give you an example. Sometimes I get woken up as if somebody's tapping me on the inside of my chest. I'm used to it, but in the middle of the night little things like that can easily become amplified in my mind. Before I know it, I've got a catastrophic conversation going on in my head, my heart is beating faster, and I'm on a spiral, a very frightening spiral. To have Jose there, someone I trust with every fibre of my body, is more than amazing, it's a gift, one she gives me night after night, day after day. Instead of staring bleakly into the darkness, with my fears all bottled up, I – she – can reset my emotions. That applies to hundreds of different scenarios that can happen anywhere, any time. I know, wherever I am in the world, whatever the time difference, whatever her commitments, she is there. Considering she has her own busy life – she is the most independent woman I have ever met – it is little short of incredible. I was lucky because I'd never known anything else but total support from her. Even so, when somebody steps up like she has, it's unbelievable. I don't know how anyone could get through what I have on their own. As it is we've become supports for one another. When one of us crumbles the other one finds the strength. It has to be that way, because if we both lost our strength the consequences don't bear thinking about.

It's a better life for Jose now that I am no longer a professional sportsman. Top-level cricketers spend many, many more nights in hotels than they do at home. Now we see a lot more of each other, although my coaching and commentary work still accounts for many a day where we see each other's faces only on a phone screen. Jose could have been forgiven for tiring of having a partner so rarely at home, but when it comes to me being an international cricketer she never wanted it any other way. She knew it was what I needed, just the same as I knew she needed her own life, to pursue her own career. She never wanted to be in the WAGs' box at a cricket match. Nothing against those who enjoy that environment, but it just wasn't her. Jose is a science teacher. And that's her to a T. She's a giving person, the kindest in the whole world, but equally she's the toughest. If I was a pupil in her class I would not want to be arguing with her! Prior to that, she worked at a charity called Teach First, which gets those with top degrees into inner city schools. Medicine or law was the more clearly defined path for her at university, with greater reward. She didn't want that. It'll embarrass her when I say this, but she wanted to make a difference. And I'm incredibly proud of that. It would doubtless have made my life easier if she was happy doing what I wanted, but what kind of relationship is it where someone makes such a one-sided sacrifice? I love the fact Jose is independent and has her own ambitions – most of which don't involve me! We rely on each other a lot, but we don't over rely on each other.

When it comes to the worries of others, there's a limit to how much I can control what's going on with myself physically, but I can control the area that those close to me have been most concerned about – how I am mentally. Again, that's down to Jose. The only time outside cricket I ever went to see a psychologist or counsellor was when I wanted to control my feelings of being anxious or nervous. I wanted a coping mechanism if my heart started misbehaving. The ECB sorted it out and I went to see a lovely woman in Derby. She was great, really helpful, and easy to talk to. But because Jose had always offered me that rock of psychological support, I felt as if I wasn't learning anything new. Instead I talked my mindset through with Jose and together we worked it out. For your wife to be your psychologist is just brilliant.

Who counsels the psychologist? Well, Jose has the most amazing family around her. The change in her life, with all the emotional turmoil that has come with it, was dropped on her in the space of minutes. Inside, she must have been really struggling. At the same time she had to be strong for me. Looking back, I don't know how she did it. All I can do is be thankful that she has such incredible people around her.

We've learnt so much about each other in the past two years. Jose is like her mum – too nice – but I always knew she had a real toughness and resilience. What I hadn't counted on was the blinding light of positivity she shone on me. I'd always thought I was the more positive one whilst Jose would analyse situations a bit more, which I sometimes perceived as negative. Here actually was a person whose inner positivity, a determination to make the very best of our new life, was extraordinary. For sure, I saw something in her that I hadn't quite realised was there.

Conversely, until the attack happened, Jose didn't truly realise what I was like. She thought everything in my life had landed on a plate – that I wasn't tough, someone who'd had to fight. Only when it looked like it was going to be taken away did she realise just what I'd invested in the life I had – thousands upon thousands of hours of training, coaching, playing, travelling, stress. Every part of me was wrapped in the game. Cricket built the foundation of who I was, and now that foundation was vanishing from beneath my feet.

That realisation of each other's hidden depths has been incredible. I – we – may not be invincible, but we know we've got the strength to get through the worst that life, and potentially death, can throw at us.

Nothing was ever going to take one of us away from the other. From early on, we both knew we'd be spending the rest of our lives together, and not long after I was out of hospital I asked Jose to marry me. I'd planned it before I got ill – I bought the ring in South Africa. I'm glad I did because the last thing I wanted it to look like was a kneejerk reaction.

I organised for me and Jose to go to her native Shropshire. I was always going to propose that summer but after everything we'd been through, why wait? We both needed a boost, something to celebrate and look forward to.

I didn't want Jose to have any clue as to my plans. However, I'd bought a magnum of champagne, which she found in the car boot. Naturally it raised suspicions.

'What are you doing with this?'

I had to think quick. 'I thought it would be nice to give your parents for being so great since everything happened.'

The night before the proposal, I told Jose's mum. She was over the moon. In the morning, just before we set off on the picnic where I'd ask the question, I told her dad. I couldn't tell him too early because I knew he couldn't keep a secret! I'm not the most traditional kind of guy so it wasn't exactly the well-worn routine of asking for a daughter's hand in marriage. It was more, 'Dennis, I'm going to ask Jose to marry me – is that OK?'

We set up the picnic in our favourite spot – the exact same place we'd had our first picnic eight years previously as teenagers. I had to propose there. Jose loves Shropshire, I love Shropshire, and we both love each other. The other option I had in mind was the beach in Perth, Western Australia – the first one was a little easier to arrange!

As we laid out the blanket and emptied the hamper, I knew for my heart's sake I couldn't get too nervous, so waiting too long for the exact right moment wasn't an option. I just did it. I got down on one knee. 'Jose, will you marry me?'

There were a few tears – more than a few actually – as we hugged. Above us on the slope some people were walking past. We asked if they could take our picture. It turned out one of them was a professional photographer – some things are just meant to be.

The wedding was a year later in the little church in Jose's village. Jose didn't do the traditional thing and be late because she didn't want me at the end of the aisle worrying – that heart thing again. That's the kind of person she is. But I had no nerves. None at all. I felt naturally chilled.

Beforehand, everybody kept telling me, 'It's going to be the best day of your life'.

'Yeah,' I'd agree, 'it is going to be a great day, but how can it match the emotion of scoring a hundred?'

As soon as I arrived at the church, I realised what they meant. All I felt was an overwhelming all-encompassing happiness. Usually the groom stays at the altar the whole time, but after the year I'd had I did things how I wanted. I didn't wait at the end of the aisle; I greeted everyone who came into the church at the door. Everybody was as happy as I'd ever seen them. It felt like there was an extra emotion in the air, as if people appreciated the value of life just that little bit more.

When Jose arrived, bang on time, she looked beyond amazing, a true vision of beauty. Here, now, in this church was everything, everyone, I ever wanted. With Jose at my side, now and forever, I could not have been happier. It was, as they had all told me, the best day of my life.

Afterwards, we retired to a marquee in Jose's uncle's garden. When it came to the speeches I had filmed mine in advance and it was shown on a screen, which in itself caused some amusement. I had to do it that way. Getting up in front of everyone was a prospect that may have prompted nervousness. Adrenalin and anxiety up your heart rate, and that was a risk, on my wedding day, I was unwilling to take. It might have put a little bit of a dampener on proceedings if I'd keeled over. I just wanted to enjoy the day, the whole beautiful experience of marrying Jose, without worrying about what was coming next, what I might have to do.

I also wanted my wedding to be an occasion full of positive thoughts about the future. I didn't want to look at something and have a reminder of what had gone. The only two England players who came to my wedding were Jonny Bairstow and Chris Woakes. Chris was my best man, one of three with Jose's brother Campbell and my old school pal Jonny Griffiths. From a cricket point of view, I deliberately wanted to keep the occasion low key to emphasise that it was truly about me and Jose and those close to us. It wasn't that I didn't want other England players there; it just felt like the wedding could quite easily turn into something it wasn't meant to be. The day was about us, not famous cricketers.

For our first dance we chose *This Will Be (An Everlasting Love)* by Natalie Cole. As it finished, I picked Jose up and swung her around. It was the sort of thing I would have done all the time before my diagnosis. As she clung to me, with a smile so wide, I looked round the dance floor. All I could see were people grinning, laughing and cheering. The love pouring out of everyone was amazing. I had the perfect wedding day marrying the perfect person.

We didn't have a proper honeymoon. We spent a couple of days in the Lake District but then came back to sort out our new home. We got the keys to the house on the Friday after we got married. It all added to the feeling of two people setting out on a new chapter together. One day hopefully we'll add another little voice to this house, and another, and another. We've always wanted a family, so the thought that our chances might be compromised by the ARVC gene was hard. Our spirits sunk when we heard there's a 50 per cent chance that if I give the dominant version of the gene to a child then they would have the genetic disposition to develop the condition. Thankfully, though, there is now a process, a little like IVF, which reduces that chance to virtually zero. Pre-implant genetic diagnosis makes it viable to test for the condition right from the start. It's a massive ray of hope for us.

In a situation like ours, where we can see only too well the effect of ARVC, no one wants to take a gamble.

When it comes to what I'll be able to do with the kids if we do have them, I try not to worry about it. My dad never really did the running round the garden stuff either because his body was so messed up with the injuries he suffered in his horse racing career. There's other ways to be a dad. It doesn't bother me so long as I can be there for them – and I can. I can do as much as I want, to a limit. One thing for sure is that our kids won't be going to boarding school. Jose is really close with her family and finds it hard to see the plus sides of distance. She's adamant our kids won't do the same as me.

We have all that, hopefully, to come. Right now, considering the upheaval, the tears, the sheer world tipped upside down-ness of the last two years, it's a beautiful thing just to have a future.

It's easy to think of my being here as being down to doctors, procedures, operations, and it is – but only to a point. In reality, Jose is my life vest. She has kept me afloat when I should have been sinking. She has brought me through nightmares, real and imagined. She has always been there – and that's how it is when you're part of each other.

Chapter 13

James (by Jose)

'Apart from anything else, Jose, you deserve something to smile about.' James's words when he proposed will stay with me always. Barely out of hospital and already he was trying to make my sun shine again.

There were times when thoughts of brightness, levity and joy seemed as remote as the panorama we were now gazing at. We'd gone from the suffocating bleakness of those endless nights in hospital to the clear pristine beauty of a spring Shropshire day … from a brick wall to a boundless future.

I never truly believed James would die, but I worried about losing him. When I felt his heart in the back of his mum's car I didn't know if he was going to make it to hospital. Then in the hospital that first night I woke up absolutely terrified, gripped by fear – 'I can't live without him.' Desperation makes you realise what you really need. It focuses you massively when you're in a space where you might lose the most important thing to you.

There were always these fleeting scares – fleeting nightmares. But I never truly thought he'd go. I wasn't going to let that happen, and never will. Whatever those horrible little voices in my head might have been saying, I knew he was a fighter. And even while the doctors were telling us terrible things about James's condition, they were also telling us that no one else had ever gone through what he had. It confirmed how strong he was. I never doubted that.

At the darkest moments in hospital, lying silently on that camp bed, I'd remember how hard it was when he was away playing cricket and I'd be on my own all through the winter. 'He's here now,' I'd console myself. 'This isn't quite how we'd have wanted it, but he's here and we're together. If I'm with him, it's all right. We're together. It's OK. He's alive. So what am I complaining about? That's all I need – for him to be alive.'

At that point I loved him more than I ever had. And that was where my real fear lay – that I'd lose him as a person. I was so afraid that the happy-go-lucky person I loved so dearly might disappear. Or at least fade. I was terrified that his character might be bruised by the heartache. It's ridiculous, I know, but my mind kept returning to a Sunday lunch we'd had that Easter, a couple of weeks before James became ill. James had always been adamant he didn't like cinnamon. Completely convinced he hated it. I knew he actually really liked it. I used to cook things with cinnamon in and he'd enjoy them, but when he found out cinnamon was among the ingredients, he'd then claim he no longer liked them. So that Sunday I made sure Mum put plenty of cinnamon in the apple pie. And I let him eat a huge slice. He asked for a second piece and I sat watching him eat it, enjoying every bite. When he'd finished, I said, 'You liked that, didn't you Jim?' And he knew what I'd done immediately. He grabbed me and tickled me so hard I could have cried. We laughed for so long about it.

My head returned to that scene again and again. It felt as if moments such as that that were over, that we could never be so carefree or occupied by such trivia again. The world felt so serious and heavy and I thought it would always be tarnished. I longed for such easy humour and untroubled times. I didn't want them during the hospital stay necessarily, but I just wanted to know that they would return. Because that's what I have with James. I've never had that in any other area of my life. Without James I take life far too seriously. So the thought of losing it broke my heart into a million pieces.

It was a fear I only ever shared with my mum. 'He won't come home a different person,' she told me, 'there's no breaking him.'

She knew the strength he had. I overheard a conversation she had with my brother during our hospital stay. Campbell commented on how remarkable James had been. 'Well,' replied my mum, 'he's the bravest person I've ever met – he took on Jose, for God's sake!' And she was right! We never did lose what we had. And he still professes to hate cinnamon to this day.

We followed James in hospital. Mad – this was happening to him, but we were all learning how to cope by taking his lead. My whole outlook on life changed by how I saw him deal with his trauma. Still to this day, we're all just following him. For James, it was never 'What do I do? How do I get round this in my head? What do I do next?' It was 'Right, this has happened. It's done. How are we going to make the best of it?' When you see someone actually doing that, it's incredible. In my head, I think that is the way you should do it. But is that even possible? No. So when you see someone deal with something in that way, you become swept up in it. You begin to realise, actually, this is the best way. It makes everything so much easier.

That approach might be taken for bravado, someone trying to make it easier for those around them, to make it seem that they were not as emotionally affected as people feared. But there was none of that with James. With him it was truly 'This is what we're doing'. There's not been one day where he hasn't just made the best of it. He's never complained. Never. He's never said 'Why has this happened to me?' He doesn't compare himself to anybody, ever. You hear about people who retire normally and can't watch cricket. James watches it and truly wants the boys to succeed. He wants the guy who took his place to get a century. There's no comparison in his head at all. No resentment. No bitterness. I don't know how he does it. I wish I could be like that. I thought so highly of James before, but I never knew the person he was.

There were times still, though, when I had to hide my desperation, my helplessness, like when James came home from his defib operation in such good spirits, so happy he hadn't had to stay overnight, only to be plunged into another nightmare of fear and pain. I think that was my most angry. James was so fragile, and had been my strength for so long, and I couldn't do anything to help him. It was the first time I felt like he might have lost a bit of his fighting spirit. That lasted for a couple of days. I too lost my positivity and felt robbed. And then he came out the other side. His confidence grew and as soon as the physical pain started to disappear, he started to reappear. 'Of course I'm taking you to Ascot, Jose!' And a couple of days later there we were. It will always be one of the best days of my life. Against all the odds he took that huge step back into life.

Apart from that tiny short period, his determination, his fighting spirit, was never bowed. He needed tests in hospital that he had to stay still for. In James's head, this was his chance to prove the doctors wrong, to turn back the narrative of this being an unstoppable illness. To James, the better he performed in the tests, the better the outcome, so the nurses would come in and he would insist on complete silence. He would shut his eyes and concentrate so hard. I would be at the end of the bed afraid to move in case I disturbed him. His face would be so concentrated, so intent on trying to stop the inevitable. On one of these occasions, I couldn't help but watch him and silently sob to myself. The tears literally rolled off my face and splashed on to the floor. I didn't even want to reach for a tissue in case I disturbed his concentration and broke his hope, shattered his dream that still existed amidst the bitter reality. When the test was over he'd open his eyes and smile so brightly. 'I did well, didn't I Jose!' You always do well.

I knew his strength. I'd seen it. But even then I'd worry he couldn't take any more. Another bombshell would fall and I'd place myself in its path to deflect it. There was a time where it was looking as if his dad Steve may have ARVC as well. His mum heard that this was a likely eventuality while James was mid-operation. She relayed this information to me. 'No,' I thought. 'Not now, not now.' I sobbed to my mum and sister that I couldn't have him hear that, it was too much. So his mum and I decided we wouldn't tell him right away. He should at least have some time to recover from the operation. When he came round from the anaesthetic, I was sat on James's bed. John Walsh came in to discuss the op and the conversation turned to his family's health.

'I'm adamant my dad doesn't have ARVC,' stated James.

In that moment I felt so sick. I didn't want to keep any secrets from him. I worried that the moment I kept something from him, he might keep something from me. And we'd already discussed that the only way we were going to make it through was to share everything. If I knew he was telling me everything then I knew he was fine when he said he was fine. And from his point of view, him sharing everything hopefully lessened the strain.

John actually looked at me in that moment and said, 'Jose, are you ok? All the colour has drained from your face.' I obviously brushed it off but that was the last of the secrets. And very luckily, it turned out his dad got the all-clear in terms of ARVC.

James's positivity would knock me sideways sometimes. The night before we met John Walsh for the definitive diagnosis, I asked how he was feeling.

'I'm really looking forward to seeing John,' he said. And that summed James up to me. He didn't mention that John was going to tell us how his life would be from then on; it was just 'I'm looking forward to seeing him'. He could focus on that. I thought, 'God!'

It was the same with his room at the hospital. It wasn't exactly a room with a view – and why should it be? It's in a hospital. But James never complained or was negative about it. His attitude was, 'At least it's got a window'. Always grateful for the little things.

Sometimes, those days in hospital feel like a different time, different people. I'm happy with that. I wouldn't want to relive some of those moments ever. Life could feel so precarious. The night he woke up sobbing after being told his life was over as he knew it – how does anybody deal with that? I would do my best to reassure him that we still had each other and always would. It was all we had. There was nothing else to hang on to.

Life totally changed at that point. I always looked at the big picture but when you're reduced to that, you're literally just living hour by hour. 'Is he all right this hour? Right, OK, I'm going to live in this hour, because I don't know what might happen in the next one.' I didn't want to think about what might happen tomorrow, I could only try to enjoy my time with him now. It helped me get through. 'If we are going to have a reduced time together, I'm going to make the best of it.' It was a way of finding a survival mechanism. I remember when someone said not to worry, something else would probably kill him first, and just thinking it was the best news ever. Odd, but true.

The day he came out, I wanted to feel real happiness but actually I found it really sad. It came from putting him back where he used to be, where he belonged, but as a different person. It didn't have the same impact in hospital, because the whole environment was different. Now, to see him back in his old environment but with a life vest on, having been through so much, and looking so fragile, made me realise how much had changed. You can't help but see your old life compared to what it has become.

At that point I suddenly felt a huge weight of responsibility. Overnight it went from knowing if there was something wrong there were doctors to help us, to now it just being me. His chest was sore, and he was asking me about symptoms, what's OK, what's normal. I didn't know. I hadn't got a clue! I'd feel his pulse, and the only reason I'd do it was so he thought I knew what I was doing – so he would be at peace. He was so nervous about his heart rate that I thought if he believed someone was in control he would settle. There were a lot of points where I felt I wanted to say something about this new us, but I didn't because I didn't want to bring him down. If James was fine, then I should be fine too.

I was worried also what might happen when the attention slowed down, when the tweets stopped coming, the letters stopped falling on the doormat. I needn't have been concerned. He had so much to focus on that when the attention slowed down, he didn't slow down with it. He was doing *Test Match Special*, appearing on *Good Morning Britain*, watching rugby – just getting back in the world again. We just followed in his slipstream. If he was doing it then we all did. He would also still upload cricket pictures. He found joy in seeing his past glories, not sadness.

Our wedding certainly allowed me something positive to think about. But there were certain points in the run-up where I couldn't help thinking, 'Why have I done this – put him in a situation of potential strain when I didn't have to? What the hell have I done? Why didn't we just get married quietly and have a party?' Again, I'd totally underestimated James. When I walked into the church he was so relaxed, hands in pockets. A friend said how much she wanted to send me a picture from the church while I was on the way because he was just standing there laughing. At that point when I saw him it truly felt like none of the past year had even happened. It couldn't have been further removed from when it had all begun.

I wish I didn't but I remember that day he left for Cambridge as clearly as I do the wedding day. He was deciding which car to go in. 'Shall I go in my Audi or my Land Cruiser?' That was the extent of our dilemmas that morning. He decided on the Land Cruiser. I didn't even say 'Good luck for the game'.

As soon as I heard James's voice on the phone that second morning, I knew something was badly wrong. 'I've got to go,' he said, and put the phone down. I burst into tears. There'd be many more in the months to come.

I texted friends in the medical profession to get some advice, but I'd already made my decision to set off home, calling him over and over again on the way. I got no reply. I didn't know it, but he was asleep in Jackson Bird's car. That wasn't great. I was thinking all kinds of things. But at the same time I had no real thought in my head that something truly terrible had happened. I was worried – because I'm a worrier – but not extremely worried. I wasn't really aware of sudden adult death. I knew about it but I wasn't about to equate it with James. We'd been together nine years and he was the fittest person I'd ever met. I always thought he was invincible.

When I finally got home, I pulled up outside and looked at myself in the mirror. I was colourless. 'Oh my God,' I thought. 'I look awful.' Subconsciously, I was obviously really scared. Even before I touched him, I could tell he was in trouble. His speech was slurring, it sounded lazy, not like him at all. He got up off the sofa and I went to feel his heart. This sounds terrible, but I almost didn't want to get anywhere near him. I couldn't feel his heart like that. I wanted to give him a hug, but I couldn't. The rate it was beating frightened me. It was awful. Horrendous. He was grey. I've never seen anything like it.

He then began crawling up the stairs, was sick, and climbed into bed. James was cold, so cold, clutching a hot water bottle to his chest. I'd never seen him like that, so childlike, vulnerable. It struck me as something so, so horrendous. When we set off to hospital I grabbed loads of coats to put over him. On the way was a roundabout that offered an opportunity to take a quicker route. James's mum took the other way. It wasn't her fault; she didn't know the roads like I do, but I was so close to screaming. The only reason I didn't was that I was trying to be calm for James, to give off this feeling that there was nothing wrong.

There was a horrible moment where I briefly touched his heart again. In my head, I was hoping so much it had gone back to normal. Instead I got that same rushing feeling. Horrible, horrible, horrible. It made me feel physically ill. It was so raw. Again I was struggling to give him a hug – 'I can't feel that'. I wasn't crying. I was too in the moment – the moment of wanting it to stop, wanting him to be better, wanting someone to help.

Wanting him to be James again. The whole emotional side of it all hadn't had an opportunity to kick in yet.

While Mum parked, James and I went to reception. I went up to the desk and the woman asked what we were there for.

'I'm here with my boyfriend,' I told her. 'He's seriously ill. His heart is beating out of his chest. He's grey.'

She couldn't actually see him because he was in the toilet being sick. She was so slow. So … slow.

'How long has he been ill? What is your connection to him?'

I was just thinking, 'You need to see him!' I was trying to make it clear that he needed to see someone straight away.

'He's being sick in the toilet right now!' It was so hard to make it clear just how serious it was. To be fair, they must have people arriving like that all the time.

Eventually, a nurse intercepted James as he came out of the toilet and took him into a little room. She put the ECG pads and wires on him and took a look at the screen. My eyes were on her, and her face was one of absolute astonishment. It was a look of 'Oh my god!'

She took James out and straight into an emergency room next door. I wasn't allowed to go through, which was when I finally started to cry. The same nurse came and sat next to me.

'We see this all the time,' she consoled me. 'Don't worry about it.'

She went off and spoke to someone, clearly thinking I couldn't hear. 'We've just had someone in here with a heart rate of 265,' she said. 'Never seen anything like it.' I started crying again. James's mum came in from the car park and found me. I told her they'd taken him through, and we sat there in complete silence. After a few moments, the medics came and got me.

'They're going to shock me,' James told me. 'I don't want them to do it.' I was thinking, 'How can you not want this to end? Shock him! Do something to him! Do anything!'

The sound of the machine in the corner was overwhelming. I can still see his face. He looked so scared – probably the only time I saw him look scared during the whole ordeal.

At that point, the drugs kicked in and brought his heart rate down naturally. 'Thank God,' I thought. 'I knew this was nothing.'

I was holding James's hand the whole time and stroking his head. I couldn't give him a hug because I had loads of coats in my hand. Loads of coats! Bloody coats! Hundreds of them!

Everything calmed down. We could still hear the noise of the heart machine. It was so lovely. So slow. It felt like one beat every thirty seconds. So nice to hear. I couldn't believe how quickly it had changed – and then he was sick everywhere. His body was just heaving. He was sitting upright with no top on. His whole body was straining.

But even then, to us it was, 'Right. OK. Off we go.'

'You're going to have to stay the night.'

For me, something changed right there and then. 'This is here to stay,' I thought. 'Life's different.' I pushed that thought out for weeks. But I knew.

James was then put in an ambulance – him in the back, me in the front – on blue lights across Nottingham. In the back, they kept telling me 'He's smiling', because I was upset. I was never upset in front of James, but as soon as he was out of sight I cried.

I never expected to move into a hospital. But there was nowhere else I wanted to be. I'd still be there now if I needed to be. I just wanted to protect him. I was so worried whenever he moved. I didn't want him to get up, didn't want him to go to the water fountain. I didn't want him anywhere away from those machines, because I was just so scared.

Every time a doctor walked in with the results of a test, my heart sank. When you're clinging on for dear life, it's easy to feel like the smallest thing is going to knock your fingers away. I tried to stay positive, telling him it was just like having a broken leg – these things happen. Inside, I was desperately trying to be as certain. In the end, any semblance of certainty turned to dust with those four letters – ARVC.

At that point for me it would take days to reach a conclusion on what I needed to do, where in my head I needed to be. And yet there was James again. He already had a plan. So black and white, as if he has an instinct. With James there was no period of self-mourning. No bitterness. Nothing. I was scared he was moving on blindly, desperate to cover up his real feelings. I was worried he was taking the easy route. To me, you need to face things to get over them. That's how I am. I thought his was an unhealthy approach, that he couldn't face the negativity. It reminded me of when his friend Alex died. I thought he wasn't facing it and he needed to. But I realise now he just doesn't dwell on things. He wasn't running away from his diagnosis. He was just hugely good at turning something terrible into something positive. He wasn't blanking it out, shutting himself off, he was dealing with it in his own way. It wasn't a case of him holding back the dam. He truly did come to terms with it in record speed. When it comes to change, he doesn't look back. It's not that he hasn't faced it; it's just that me facing it would take years and him facing it took twenty-four hours. He faces it and doesn't hold on to any of the negatives. I don't know any other person in the whole world who could do that.

I look at James now and two thoughts go round and round in my mind: 'He's still alive, and he's happy.' But it's an alive and happy with conditions. The main condition is we can never forget for one minute.

Early on, I remember us disagreeing over something. I was across the table and James suddenly stopped. I could see his shirt moving. I felt so guilty. But things like that are with us all the time. Now I'd be more confident that a situation like that wasn't going to turn into something worse. Back then, any minor incident felt potentially catastrophic.

As time went on I knew he needed to get his lifestyle back. Because if there's one thing I've learned from all this it's that you've got to live. I can't just keep him at home wrapped in cotton wool, as much as I'd prefer it. At first when he started going away coaching or working, I was pleased. Antigua made it rather more difficult. I was stood in a classroom, kids at the door, wanting to come in, and my husband was on the phone saying goodbye because he thought he was about to die. That was awful, really awful. I was in proper shock after that, more so than at any other point.

People wonder whether experiences like that have taken their toll on me. But actually, rather than damaged me, the entire experience with James has helped me mentally. Beforehand, I'd never have believed anybody could get through something like this without struggling. But to watch James do it has made me see that is an option. It has helped me. I think I am mentally stronger now. I've got things in perspective. Obviously, I still worry, but as a person I'm a lot more positive. I enjoy my life way more.

I always remember that while times were tough we never felt the true desperation that others have to face. We were, and are, lucky. So unbelievably lucky. We're sad from time to time, sure, but we've always had somewhere to turn – to each other. I can't imagine the pain of the wives and husbands, mothers and fathers, sons and daughters, who hear the letters ARVC for the first time when it's too late. I can't ask for anything more than being able to spend my life with James. I have that. So I class us both as truly lucky. We've had something happen in our lives that has made us realise how good we have it. And what we have is too special to tarnish with the longing for things that we're never going to get back.

Life ends at some point. No matter what age, it ends. If you've spent it looking back, what do you have then?

Chapter 14

Now

I'm not scared of life – I'm scared of my heart. I'm scared because I know the extent of its potential to cause me harm. A heart condition isn't a broken arm. You can't put it in plaster and wait for it to mend. It is there all the time – and it isn't shy of issuing a reminder.

I am absolutely guaranteed several more potentially traumatic events. My defib lasts for eight to ten years in terms of battery. The lead that travels from the defib into my heart lasts fifteen to twenty. With a normal life expectancy, I'm looking at five or six defib changes and two or three lead changes. Every time there is a small risk of introducing infection and complication.

But despite having seen the fragility of life in all its inglorious detail, I can't allow that image to dominate who I am. Why accept negative emotion? Much better to be positive.

If I'd had a heart condition when I was eleven, my mum would have wrapped me in cotton wool and I'd never have done anything. Instead I've travelled the world, played international sport, and met some amazing people.

Had it been discovered when I was nineteen, something similar would have happened. I'd have been advised to stop playing cricket and I'd have missed out on all those incredible experiences.

Because of that, people believe me to be at the centre of some great philosophical paradox – the fact that had the condition been active and detected when I was nineteen I would have missed out on my cricket career, but alternatively I might not have nearly died.

I don't care. I really don't. Clearly, I would rather not be in the position I am, but in my head I know I've had the best possible outcome. I made it as an international cricketer, with the acclaim and recognition that went with it. Give it up at nineteen and I wouldn't have been James Taylor the cricketer, I'd have been some bloke who was half decent at cricket when he was younger who had to retire.

Equally, I know I shouldn't be here. But again I look at that as a positive. I've battled through something that kills 80 per cent of those it afflicts. I've survived six marathons on the bounce. If that doesn't give you confidence in your physical and mental strength, then nothing will. That old me hasn't died, I've just had to make a transition. I used to be super confident in my image and my body. Now I'm more confident in myself but much less confident in my physicality.

Right from the word go in hospital, I took so much from the fact I had survived. Why be negative about what's gone when you have still got the greatest gift of all in your hands? I will always look at how incredibly fortunate I am. When the doctor said to me 'You can't play cricket anymore. You can't exercise', I broke down. When he then said to me 'If it's any consolation, in 80 per cent of people ARVC is found in post-mortem', my world didn't seem quite so bad.

I'm constantly reminded of how lucky I am by the messages I receive. I've had hundreds of emails, letters, messages on social media, either asking me for help, or telling me how I'm helping others through my positivity. I had a letter recently from a parent whose son had died in his sleep. I read it and then handed it to Jose. It was a blunt reminder of what we've got – and what so many others haven't. A dozen teenagers every week die from conditions related to mine, normally while playing sport. Make no mistake; I really am one of the lucky ones. Hopefully, when it comes to cardiac care, I can help there be more lucky ones by spreading a message of education and hope as an ambassador for the British Heart Foundation.

It's all too easy to forget also that there are families mourning young cricketers who would give anything to have their loved ones still with them, with or without a career. Phil Hughes was playing for Middlesex when I made my debut first class hundred. I remember him throwing grapes on the wicket on a length after tea! I was with England in Colombo, just getting on the team bus, when we heard the news that he'd died. Some of the guys closer to Phil – Steve Finn, for instance, and Moeen Ali, who'd both played with him – were understandably really cut up. We all put our bats out for him in Sri Lanka.

Tom Maynard was another taken tragically young. I'd roomed with him in the early days when we were in the ECB camps at Loughborough. He was a funny guy, an entertainer, and I loved just listening to him tell stories. He was seriously talented and would undoubtedly have played for England. I couldn't take it in when I heard he'd died. Stuart Broad rang me just as I was leaving my apartment. I stood in the car park listening in disbelief. I'd just been on tour with him to Bangladesh with the Lions. And now he was gone.

Perspective is a great thing. I might not have my life as it was. But I still have everything. Arrhythmogenic right ventricular cardiomyopathy – those words are attached to me forever. But at least I'm still here.

The last two years has taught me a lot. I've had a fast and occasionally brutal education in how to survive in my new physical state. The risks don't dominate my thoughts anymore. The dos and don'ts are increasingly ingrained. ARVC is a constant background noise. At times it can loom loud, on other occasions it plays its discordant tune more gently. The hardest thing for me is witnessing its effect on those around me. What's happened to me has caused an incredible strain on others. My family aren't ones for a DMC (deep and meaningful conversation) – that's probably what shaped my toughness and determination - but that's not to say they don't care. My mum worries still. Any time I have to go to hospital for a check-up she wants to come. She doesn't want me to be on my own. I've never seen my dad get upset but my mum has. I know it hit my dad harder than he gave away at the time, and the strange and ugly comparisons between the loss of his sporting career and mine are not lost on either of us.

More pertinently, worries and fears about ARVC in our family go much further than me. ARVC is a genetic condition. It was never likely to have snaked its way into only my DNA. Tests have confirmed that to be the case. The ARVC gene has been found in my mum, my auntie, and potentially, my cousin. The positive side is they at least now have the knowledge and can take measures to deal with it. Forewarned, as they say, is forearmed. For my mum's part, she laughs her own situation off. As she reminds me, the last bit of exercise she did was when she tried to beat the 9-year-old me at tennis. But it doesn't lessen the long-term and deeply unsettling impact that ARVC has had across the family.

We all have to adapt and change, and thankfully that's something I've always been good at. In my sporting life I had coping mechanisms in place to deal with stress, generally by turning it to my advantage, to the extent I would thrive on it to make me stronger and drive me forward. Now, in my new life, there's a horrible irony that the very emotion I used to thrive on is the one thing I avoid at all costs. I absolutely hate it. That clearly places limitations on how I move forward. I've had business opportunities mentioned but I've always quashed such conversations before they got going. I don't want to lead anybody on. I'm not interested in doing something I don't know anything about at the moment. I've had challenges enough recently to be taking any more on board! There's always an incentive to make money, but I would happily sacrifice that money to have a less stressful life. I've got a focused edge but in a different way.

When I got out of hospital, I said I wanted to do things that I knew and enjoyed. Coaching definitely ticked those two boxes. It was always something

I thought I'd be decent at, and fortunately others in the game backed my judgement as I was asked to work with the Nottinghamshire Academy and Nottinghamshire second team, and then as Northamptonshire batting coach, before the job came up with England U-19s.

Coaching is a very different skill set from playing. It's about the player first and foremost, whereas as a batsman it was always about me. From the start that appealed. I liked the fact that my outlook had to turn 180 degrees; I loved the psychology of it. Early on I was thinking on my feet, but I had a good base knowledge from learning from the best – Steve, Pridge, and then on to Boony, Ramps, Thorpe, Moores and beyond. I knew from their coaching the approach I needed to take, that I needed to be honest and open and assess early on what makes each player perform to their best. Being a man manager is the biggest thing for any coach. The U-19s is a challenge from that perspective because there are so many different characters in that age group, some are more mature than others, and they're learning all the time. But I was always hyper-aware of what other people were thinking in my time as a player, and that was something I took into the coaching environment. I look at these players and recognise my own insecurities from when I was starting out. I put myself back in their shoes. I try to live their lives and envisage their dreams. In many ways, young players are so different, and yet they all want the same. I hope that, for now at least, they can relate to me because I'm a similar generation.

How far coaching will take me, I'm unsure. At the moment I just want to improve, that is all. I could be interested in taking it further in a few years, but having just come out of a near death experience I'm a little too selfish at the moment.

Some wonder if it presents a difficulty being in a cricket environment when I'm denied the pleasure of picking up a bat anymore. I did actually have a bat for five minutes with a mate, and I did some filming against a bowling machine, and I loved it. It was like I hadn't been anyway. But it didn't bother me when I put that bat back down, because I know I can't come out of retirement. Physically, I can't do it. Inevitably, I'd have another heart attack. That makes walking away a lot easier. Yes, in an ideal world I'd still be playing for England. I'd be back off the plane to Australia having just dispatched Starc, Cummins and the rest to the boundary boards of the SCG to cap off an Ashes-winning contribution. But that doesn't mean I sit at home dreaming of it. ARVC put a full stop on it. My mum definitely thinks I should be in the side when she watches England, but I don't. You have to realise honestly where you're at in life, and for me, coming to terms with the end of my cricketing career, while upsetting, was vitally important. I know I should have played more for England but I can't. I definitely can't. That's a lot different from saying I could have played a lot more for England but I'm not because they've picked someone else.

I might be able to play a bit of club cricket, but why would I risk doing that on such a small stage? The thought of having another incident, of being scared witless again, is horrible. I get scared enough in everyday life – the mere thought of my heart getting out of control is scary – without adding to it by putting myself in an unnecessary position.

I have to find fulfilment in other ways, and perhaps the most unexpected has been broadcasting. When I was imagining what Nasser and co were saying about me as I made my way towards that century against the Aussies at Old Trafford, I wasn't expecting to be up there in the commentary box myself quite so quickly. It wasn't something I'd ever really thought of getting into, but Luke was always keen. He thought I'd be a good fit. He probably thought it would be a change for someone else to have to listen to my opinions. I was a little bit reluctant because it was the unknown. At that point, in the wake of what had happened, I didn't want to do things that were out of my comfort zone. I didn't want to challenge myself. But Luke pushed me and I started doing some overnight punditry for Sky, the benefit being for them I had only recently left the England setup and so was able to add my own unique insight. There were nerves, but I reminded myself I had spent my whole life walking into new challenges, new teams. Yet again I was relating my current life to that of a cricketer. In fact, post-retirement, the way I've conducted myself in pretty much every new environment, dealing with different characters, different workplace cultures, has all come from sport.

Throughout my life people had always told me I could speak, even if I might not have believed it at the time, and when I was actually in front of the camera I found the words came quite easily. Early in the piece I found myself thinking, 'Hang on, I'm enjoying this!' And I loved the Sky suits! The downside was the 1.00 am starts. The upside is I now find getting up at 3.00 am for a flight a piece of cake.

From the off, I decided I wanted to be a pundit passionate about the sport. Someone who has enthusiasm for cricket, rather than sprays criticism for the sake of it, or who resents change. If I'm still in the commentary box in ten years' time, I don't want to be one of those pundits constantly using the phrase 'In my day'. I never want to be the resident curmudgeon.

I took that ethos with me to *Test Match Special*, where right from the start I found an incredibly welcoming group of people keen to have a laugh and a joke, which automatically settled me down. It genuinely felt like they wanted me to be there and had a real desire to help me get better. Being around such eloquent individuals, people who really know the flexibility of language and the power of the word, made me realise early on that my vocabulary has to improve – I might have to read a few more books – but at the moment I'm fortunate in that at least I don't have to think too much about what's happening in front of me because I'm still close to the game. The longer it goes on, the more research I'll have to do. I don't balk at that – always I'm striving to get better. Even when I'm not on air myself, I'll listen, trying to pick up ways of improving, be it elements of descriptiveness or when to use humour to make a point. Being on live radio makes you focus – and quickly. Silence is no good to anybody and neither is just messing about. *TMS* has a fun side to it, but I'm not there to do a Blowers and start talking about pigeons. My role is to analyse performance, the technical side of the game, and then have a bit of fun if it comes about. The more I do *TMS*, hopefully the sharper I'll be in making a point.

What I hope more than anything is that my love of the game comes across. I think it does, simply because *TMS* encourages it in me. I can honestly say that for me it is the next best thing to playing. A little bonus is that it also allows me to stay in touch with many of my former teammates. Last winter, during the Ashes series, before I went out to commentate on the one day games, Jonny Bairstow sent me a message: 'Great,' he said, 'it's going to be just like the old times.'

I know it can be frowned upon, but it doesn't bother me that I've gone straight from the dressing room to the commentary box. People suspect, especially if you still have friendships in the pavilion, it can hold you back from what you really want to say. To me the benchmark is my not minding giving an opinion of someone so long as I would say it to their face. That player might then question my opinion, but so long as I can back it up with evidence, and show that I'm not talking a load of rubbish, I'm happy. I have already been in situations where current players have challenged me on something I've said. My response is simple: 'Tell me it's not true.' As long as I can justify what I've said, I'm happy. Some people say things just to make headlines. I don't want to be one of them. I want to be known as someone who gives an honest opinion. That way, if someone questions my view, I can come back to them with an answer, rather than being shown up as making statements for the sake of it.

TMS is another shining example of the virtues of surrounding yourself with amazing people. I'm so glad I had such an incredible support network around me for cricket, because then when I was ill, that same solid foundation of love, goodwill and positivity supported me in a much bigger battle. Without them I just don't know where I would be. They helped me through the toughest of tough innings to be not out at the end.

Along the way I learned the value of talking about my situation. It's one of the main reasons I wanted to write this book. In hospital, Jose and I were adamant we could turn my experience on its head and use it as a force for good. Maybe we might offer a ray of hope for those in a similar situation. Perhaps we could show others that ARVC isn't the end, it's just the beginning of something else. We also wanted to illustrate the value of being open, of talking about the future rather than mourning the past – and that applies to people in all kinds of circumstances.

I'm always amazed by how my story has helped others. Last winter, a chap in Australia I'd never met drove four hours from Canberra to Sydney to have a round of golf with me. He told me it was the first time in six years he'd looked forward to something. As we played, he revealed how he'd tried to take his own life. When he heard about me being ill he was devastated, but then, he explained, he saw my positivity, which inspired him to move forward with his own life and not dwell on the past. It's both amazing and humbling to influence someone's path like that.

I too am learning all the time. Beforehand, I was never an overly emotional person. I was incredibly good at blocking things out, just pulling up the shutters on anything of that nature. Utterly ruthless. Why let emotion in? It's only going to keep something more important out. Now, with all that's happened, I can see the value in expressing that side of myself. I understand how necessary, vital even, it is to have that release. Honesty is the bedrock of my life. I don't want there to be a hidden side. My condition has definitely been the catalyst to a more emotional me. It's funny. If I cry, Jose cries, and then I cry even more!

I could have disappeared from cricket, from life, from myself, had I raised the emotional barriers like I have in the past. Where once was James Taylor there would now be a shadow. I don't want to live as a grey silhouette of my former self. I want to shine brightly, for myself and all around me. Why be a closed book when you can throw open your pages to everyone? Why see ARVC as a full stop when it's the next chapter of the story? Why add yourself to the shelf marked 'History' when there's a whole new exciting future ahead?

Yes, I have scars, but because of that new honesty they are physical not mental. You can see the scars on my arms where the cannulas went in, on my chest where they opened me up and fitted the defib, but if you could look inside my head you would see none – nothing. At every turn, when those mental wounds have threatened to appear, I've had the backing of the most amazing people – friends, family, players, colleagues, and perhaps most remarkably of all, strangers. Even now I receive letters of support from people I don't know any more than you do. I find that truly incredible, and I am hugely grateful. For people to invest that time and effort in me is amazing. I just hope that I too, with my story, can offer some support to others.

It's odd to use the phrase 'Looking back' when you're twenty-eight. I never imagined it would be something I'd be doing, and it still takes a little bit of getting used to. Ultimately, I will never know what I might have achieved on the cricket pitch. Equally, that can never be my focus. Yes, occasionally, I feel an echo of sadness for what I've lost, but, as time has gone on, those echoes have become more distant. Instead I have taken the positivity of spirit I had as a player and translated it into my new life. I'm backing myself to be a decent person – a better version of James Taylor.

People always said I was a never say die character. They were right.

Acknowledgments

Mum, Dad, and Sarah – I know this can't have been easy for you. Thank you for being so strong when I really needed you. My whole life you've built me into a person who can deal with the most challenging of events.

Bridget and Dennis – from nursing my hangovers in the early years to being by my bedside when times got tough, you've always made me part of your family. You are two of the nicest people I've ever met.

Campbell and Libby – I'm so grateful for having gained an older brother and a little sister. You made me smile when I was at my lowest.

John Walsh and Tim Robinson – you are the true heroes of this world. You and all the staff who looked after me are the world's best. Aside from being brilliant doctors, you're great blokes who I'm glad to have met. You've made things so much easier for me.

Luke – I don't know where I'd be without you. Thanks for being a mate and an unbelievable agent. You took a lot of the worry out of my hands and gave me a future when I thought I'd lost everything.

The Schofields – you are like another family to me. Thanks so much for your time over the years and teaching me so much of what I know in cricket.

Pridge and Boony – you guys were instrumental in getting me to where I was in the game. The time you gave up for me was phenomenal and I've always appreciated it. I'll never forget all the hours we spent in those indoor schools together.

John Woodhouse – thank you for your patience and skill in allowing me to tell my story as I wanted. I feel fortunate to have worked with such an amazing writer as you.

Finally, to everyone who visited me in hospital and to all the thousands of people who wrote to me or sent me messages on social media; your love made such a difference. Thank you. You got me through.

James Taylor Career Statistics

James William Arthur Taylor, born Nottingham, 6 January 1990.

Right-hand bat; leg break bowler.

Wisden Schools Cricketer of the Year 2008.

Cricket Writers' Club Young Cricketer of the Year 2009.

Leicestershire 2008-11; cap 2009.

Nottinghamshire 2012-16; cap 2012.

TEST MATCH CAREER RECORD

	M	I	NO	HS	Runs	Avge	100	50	Ct
2012 to 2015-16	7	13	1	76	312	26.00	–	2	7

Match list

Opponent	Venue	Date	1st Inns	2nd Inns	Res
v South Africa	Leeds	2-6 Aug 2012	34 B	DNB	Drawn
v South Africa	Lord's	16-20 Aug 2012	10 Ct	4 RO	Lost
v Pakistan	Sharjah	1-5 Nov 2015	76 Ct	2 Ct	Lost
v South Africa	Durban	26-30 Dec 2015	70 Ct	42 St	Won
v South Africa	Cape Town	2-6 Jan 2016	0 Ct	27 Ct	Drawn
v South Africa	Johannesburg	14-16 Jan 2016	7 Ct	2 NO	Won
v South Africa	Centurion	22-26 Jan 2016	14 Ct	24 Ct	Lost

LIMITED-OVERS INTERNATIONAL CAREER RECORD

	M	I	NO	HS	Runs	Avge	100	50	Ct	S/R
2011 to 2015-16	27	26	5	101	887	42.23	1	7	7	80.12

Match list

Opponent	Venue	Date	Score	Balls	Res
v Ireland	Dublin	25 Aug 2011	1 Ct	8	Won
v Ireland	Dublin	3 Sep 2013	25 B	42	Won
v Sri Lanka	Colombo, RPS	7 Dec 2014	90 Ct	109	Lost
v Sri Lanka	Pallekele	10-11 Dec 2014	68 Ct	90	Won
v Sri Lanka	Pallekele	13 Dec 2014	10 B	12	Lost
v Sri Lanka	Colombo, RPS	16 Dec 2014	2 Ct	4	Lost
v Australia	Sydney	16 Jan 2015	0 LBW	2	Lost
v India	Brisbane	20 Jan 2015	56 NO	63	Won
v Australia	Hobart	23 Jan 2015	5 Ct	14	Lost
v India	Perth	30 Jan 2015	82 Ct	122	Won
v Australia	Perth	1 Feb 2015	4 Ct	18	Lost
v Australia (WC)	Melbourne	14 Feb 2015	98 NO	90	Lost
v New Zealand (WC)	Wellington	20 Feb 2015	0 B	2	Lost
v Scotland (WC)	Christchurch	23 Feb 2015	17 St	26	Won
v Sri Lanka (WC)	Wellington	1 Mar 2015	25 Ct	26	Lost
v Bangladesh (WC)	Adelaide	9 Mar 2015	1 Ct	4	Lost
v Afghanistan (WC)	Sydney	13 Mar 2015	8 NO	20	Won
v Ireland (captain)	Dublin	8 May 2015	DNB	–	No res
v Australia	Southampton	3 Sep 2015	49 B	51	Lost
v Australia	Lord's	5 Sep 2015	43 Ct	57	Lost
v Australia	Manchester	8 Sep 2015	101 Ct	114	Won
v Australia	Leeds	11 Sep 2015	41 Ct	42	Won
v Australia	Manchester	13 Sep 2015	12 Ct	18	Lost
v Pakistan	Abu Dhabi	11 Nov 2015	60 Ct	82	Lost
v Pakistan	Abu Dhabi	13 Nov 2015	9 NO	8	Won
v Pakistan	Sharjah	17 Nov 2015	67 NO	69	Won
v Pakistan	Dubai, DSC	20 Nov 2015	13 Ct	14	Won

FIRST-CLASS CAREER RECORD

Debut v Worcestershire, at Worcester, on 23-26 April 2008, scoring 8.

Final game v Cambridge MCCU, at Cambridge, on 5-7 April 2016, scoring 10.

	M	I	NO	HS	Runs	Avge	100	50	Ct
Leicestershire 2008	4	5	–	51	64	12.80	–	1	4
Leicestershire 2009	17	28	7	207*	1207	57.47	3	6	9
MCC in UAE 2009-10	1	2	–	39	39	19.50	–	–	1
Leics & Eng L 2010	18	29	4	206*	1095	43.80	3	4	15
England A in WI 2010-11	6	10	1	186	527	58.55	1	2	6
Leics & Eng L 2011	17	32	3	237	1602	55.24	3	10	13
Notts, Eng A & Eng 2012	18	28	4	163*	875	36.45	3	1	10
Notts, Sx & Eng L 2013	18	25	3	204*	1079	49.04	3	5	9
England A 2013-14	5	9	2	242*	459	65.57	1	2	4
Nottinghamshire 2014	15	28	2	126	992	38.15	1	8	7
Nottinghamshire 2015	13	23	2	291	1078	51.33	2	6	6
Eng in SA 2015-16	5	9	1	70	201	25.12	–	1	7
Eng in UAE 2015-16	1	2	–	70	76	38.00	–	1	–
Nottinghamshire 2016	1	1	–	10	10	10.00	–	–	–
Leicestershire	53	89	14	237	3689	49.18	9	18	40
Nottinghamshire	60	99	10	291	3745	42.07	7	20	29
Sussex	1	1	1	121*	121	–	1	–	1
MCC	1	2	–	39	39	19.50	–	–	1
England Lions	16	26	3	242*	1385	60.21	3	7	11
England †	8	14	1	76	327	25.15	–	2	9
Total	139	231	29	291	9306	46.06	20	47	91

† Total includes one match that was not a Test.

First-Class Centuries

Match	Venue	Date	Score	Balls
Leics v Middlesex	Southgate	28 Apr-1 May 2009	122 NO	197
Leics v Surrey	The Oval	31 Jul-3 Aug 2009	207 NO	329
Leics v Essex	Chelmsford	26-29 Aug 2009	112 NO	214
Leics v Middlesex	Leicester	29 May-1 Jun 2010	206 NO	271
Leics v Middlesex	Lord's	9-12 Aug 2010	106 NO	230
Leics v Northamptonshire	Northampton	13-16 Sep 2010	156 Ct	316
England Lions v Barbados	Bridgetown	11-14 Feb 2011	186 Ct	417
Leics v Loughborough MCCU	Leicester	20-22 Apr 2011	237 Ct	296
Leics v Sri Lanka A	Leicester	20-23 July 2011	168 NO	247
Leics v Glamorgan	Colwyn Bay	17-20 Aug 2011	127 NO	280
Notts v Loughborough MCCU	Nottingham	1-3 Apr 2012	101 NO	124
England Lions v West Indians	Northampton	10-13 May 2012	118 Ct	179
Notts v Sussex	Nottingham	27-30 Jul 2012	163 NO	265
Notts v Derbyshire	Derby	24-27 Apr 2013	112 Ct	282
Notts v Sussex	Nottingham	22-25 Jun 2013	204 NO	358
Sussex v Australians	Hove	26-28 Jul 2013	121 NO	253
England Lions v Sri Lanka A	Dambulla	19-22 Feb 2014	242 NO	339
Notts v Sussex	Nottingham	15-18 Sep 2014	126 Ct	189
Notts v Sussex	Hove	19-21 Jul 2015	291 Ct	385
Notts v Warwickshire	Birmingham	14-17 Sep 2015	164 LBW	260

James Taylor bowled thirty-eight overs in first class cricket, but failed to take any wickets.

LIST-A CAREER RECORD
Debut, Leicestershire v Essex, at Leicester, on 20 July 2008, did not bat.

Final game, England XI v South Africa A, at Kimberley, on 30 January 2016, scoring 116.

	M	I	NO	HS	Runs	Avge	100	50	Ct
Leicestershire 2008	4	2	1	43*	80	80.00	-	-	-
Leicestershire 2009	15	14	2	101	556	46.33	1	3	-
Eng L in UAE 2009-10	3	3	-	61	64	21.33	-	1	1
Leics & Eng L 2010	14	14	5	103*	450	50.00	1	3	4
Leics & Eng L 2011	12	11	1	111	635	63.50	3	3	3
England in Ireland 2011	1	1	-	1	1	1.00	-	-	-
Eng L in Ban 2011-12	5	5	1	65*	105	26.25	-	1	-
Eng L in SL 2011-12	5	5	-	41	96	19.20	-	-	2
Nottinghamshire 2012	8	8	2	115*	385	64.16	1	2	1
Eng L in Aus 2012-13	6	6	1	79	229	45.80	-	2	1
Notts & Eng L 2013	16	16	6	108	775	77.50	2	4	3
England in Ireland 2013	1	1	-	25	25	25.00	-	-	-
Notts & Eng L 2014	11	11	3	146*	586	73.25	4	1	4
England in SL 2014-15	4	4	-	90	170	42.50	-	2	1
England in NZ 2014-15	3	3	-	25	42	14.00	-	-	-
England in Aus 2014-15	8	8	3	98*	254	50.80	-	3	4
England in Ireland 2015	1	-	-	-	-	-	-	-	-
Notts & England 2015	14	14	3	109	647	58.81	2	3	5
England in UAE 2015-16	4	4	2	67*	149	74.50	-	2	1
England in S Af 2015-16	1	1	-	116	116	116.00	1	-	-
Leicestershire	40	36	7	103*	1451	50.03	3	9	4
Nottinghamshire	37	37	12	146*	1815	72.59	6	10	12
England Lions	31	31	6	111	1096	43.84	4	4	7
England †	28	27	5	116	1003	45.59	2	7	7
Total	136	131	30	146*	5365	53.11	15	30	30

† *Total includes one match that was not an international fixture.*

List-A Centuries

Match	Venue	Date	Score	Balls
Leics v Worcestershire	Worcester	12 May 2009	101 NO	109
Leics v Warwickshire †	Leicester	25 July 2010	103 NO	95
Leics v Warwickshire	Birmingham	1 May 2011	101 B	86
England Lions v Sri Lanka A	Worcester	12 Aug 2011	106 Ct	120
England Lions v Sri Lanka A	Northampton	16 Aug 2011	111 Ct	132
Notts v Hampshire	Southampton	31 May 2012	115 NO	77
Notts v Northamptonshire	Northampton	5 May 2013	108 Ct	102
England Lions v Bangladesh A	Taunton	22 Aug 2013	106 NO	100
England Lions v Sri Lanka A	Worcester	11 Aug 2014	103 NO	114
Notts v Middlesex	Lord's	14 Aug 2014	100 NO	55
Notts v Derbyshire	Nottingham	26 Aug 2014	146 NO	154
Notts v Durham	Chester-le-St	6 Sep 2014	114 Ct	112
Notts v Kent	Nottingham	17 Aug 2015	109 Ct	111
England v Australia	Manchester	8 Sep 2015	101 Ct	114
England XI v South Africa A	Kimberley	30 Jan 2016	116 Ct	116

† James Taylor took four wickets in the same match, dismissing Neil Carter, Rikki Clarke, Chris Woakes and Ant Botha, to finish with match figures of four for 61. His only other wicket in List-A cricket came in his next game, on 8 August, when he dismissed Joe Denly of Kent.

Nottinghamshire won the Yorkshire Bank 40 competition in 2013, beating Glamorgan by 87 runs in the final on 21 September at Lord's, with James Taylor scoring 22.

TWENTY20 CAREER RECORD
Debut, Leicestershire v Derbyshire, at Derby, on 22 June 2008, scoring 22.

Final game, Nottinghamshire v Durham, at Chester-le-Street, on 17 July 2015, scoring 37.

	M	I	NO	HS	Runs	Avge	100	50	Ct
Leicestershire 2008	3	2	–	22	32	16.00	–	–	–
Leicestershire 2009	10	10	3	41*	205	29.28	–	–	2
Leicestershire 2010	14	14	3	62*	407	37.00	–	4	5
Leicestershire 2011	18	15	6	53	342	38.00	–	1	6
Leics in India 2011-12	2	2	1	56*	67	67.00	–	1	–
Eng L in Ban 2011-12	2	2	–	43	71	35.50	–	–	1
Nottinghamshire 2012	8	5	2	45	127	42.33	–	–	1
Nottinghamshire 2013	9	9	3	54	196	32.66	–	1	5
Nottinghamshire 2014	13	12	4	52*	272	34.00	–	1	5
Nottinghamshire 2015	12	11	3	38*	253	31.62	–	–	7
Leicestershire	47	43	13	62*	1053	35.10	–	6	13
Nottinghamshire	42	37	12	54	848	33.92	–	2	18
England Lions	2	2	–	43	71	35.50	–	–	1
Total	91	82	25	62*	1972	34.59	–	8	32

Twenty20 Half-Centuries

Match	Venue	Date	Score	Balls
Leics v Yorkshire	Leicester	20 Jun 2010	60 Ct	42
Leics v Lancashire	Leicester	25 Jun 2010	61 Ct	37
Leics v Yorkshire	Leeds	27 Jun 2010	62 NO	28
Leics v Nottinghamshire	Leicester	4 Jul 2010	56 NO	38
Leics v Derbyshire	Leicester	8 July 2011	53 Ct	31
Leics v Trinidad & Tobago	Hyderabad	20 Sep 2011	56 NO	47
Notts v Durham	Nottingham	19 Jul 2013	54 Ct	43
Notts v Yorkshire	Nottingham	28 Jun 2014	52 NO	38

James Taylor took two wickets in T20 cricket, again in successive games: he dismissed Adam Lyth of Yorkshire on 25 May 2009, and Chris Rogers of Derbyshire on 28 May 2009.

Leicestershire won the Friends Life T20 competition in 2011, beating Somerset by 18 runs in the final on 27 August at Edgbaston, with James Taylor scoring 18 not out.